IMM
An Introduction

IMMUNOASSAY
An Introduction

by

Ray Edwards

*Director, North East Thames Region Immunoassay Unit
St. Bartholomew's Hospital London*

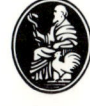

WILLIAM HEINEMANN MEDICAL BOOKS
London

First published in 1985 by William Heinemann Medical Books,
23, Bedford Square, London WC1B 3HH

© 1985 Ray Edwards

ISBN: O-433-08165-1

Typeset by Tradespools Ltd, Frome and
printed in Great Britain by The Alden Press, Oxford

CONTENTS

Chapter

1. Historical Development of Immunoassays   1
2. Basic Concepts in Immunoassay   12
3. Radioimmunoassay   24
4. Immunoradiometric Assay   41
5. Antibodies: Polyclonal and Monoclonal   55
6. Enzyme Labelled Immunoassay Methods   74
7. Fluorescent Labelled Immunoassay   87
8. Luminescent Labelled Immunoassays   100
9. Immunoprecipitation Assays   111
10. Particle and Agglutination Immunoassays   124
11. Comparison, Application and Enhancement   139

Index   159

CHAPTER ONE

Historical Development of Immunoassays

Introduction

The 1960s and the 1970s have witnessed an increasing interest in immunoassay techniques. Today, immunoassays enjoy an almost unprecedented popularity as methods of choice for quantitation. They have permeated many branches and disciplines of scientific investigation, especially in the biologically related subjects. Not only has the use of immunoassays proliferated, but also the variety and type. There are immunoassays using a variety of detection systems, such as radioisotopic measurement, fluorescence, agglutination, precipitation and enzyme colour reactions. There are assays carried out in solutions or in gels; with liquid-phase reagents or with solid-phase reagents; with monoclonal antibodies or polyclonal antibodies; and many other variations proliferating around a central theme. The expanding field of immunoassay methods seems to have offered to the experienced assayist almost unlimited opportunities for individual expression. On the other hand, the beginner has to choose from a vast array of techniques, each with, it seems, innumerable modifications. The choice is not made any easier by many extravagant claims and counter claims put forward by the various interested parties.

Acronyms

A further source of confusion for the beginner is the widespread practice of using acronyms. The growth in the number of acronyms has been as fertile as the growth in diversity of techniques. It starts, very reasonably, with RIA for radioimmunoassay and FIA for fluorescent immunoassay, developing through IRMAs (immunoradiometric assays) and ELISAs (enzyme labelled immunosorbent assays) to the current startling display of PACIAs, SIAs, ARIAs, SRIDs, NIIAs, IFMAs, LIAs, RASTs, PRISTs, SOPHIAs, PICRIAs, USERIAs and so on. On one hand, techniques have been multiplying through modifications and amendments, giving rise to a proliferation of methods, and, on the other hand, the titles have been contracting into forms yielding almost total anonymity. All of which has compounded to produce for the beginner, a bewildering and confusing choice.

In practice, the diversity usually arises not from 'artistic' individuality, but from the particular need of a specific application. A systematic and objective approach will reveal the underlying principles and indicate the most appropriate technique for the particular application in mind. As an introduction to the subject, it is useful to consider aspects of the historical development of the now almost ubiquitous immunoassay.

The Significance of Immunoassay Development

It would be difficult to deny that the publication of the first radioimmunoassay (RIA) by Berson and Yalow in 1960 was a most significant event. Indeed, many brief accounts of the development of immunoassays often imply that it was the beginning for immunoassay methods. However, a more discriminating scrutiny of the published literature would soon reveal that this was certainly not the case. Nonetheless, the publication of Berson and Yalow did arouse considerable interest, particularly amongst those actively pursuing research in the field of endocrinology. The reasons for this interest are worth noting as they have a direct bearing on subsequent developments and successful adoption of immunoassay methods in general. In brief, the published RIA method that attracted so much interest appeared to offer the following list of potential advantages:

       1) Sensitivity
       2) Specificity
       3) Simplicity
       4) Universal application

Historical Development of Immunoassays 3

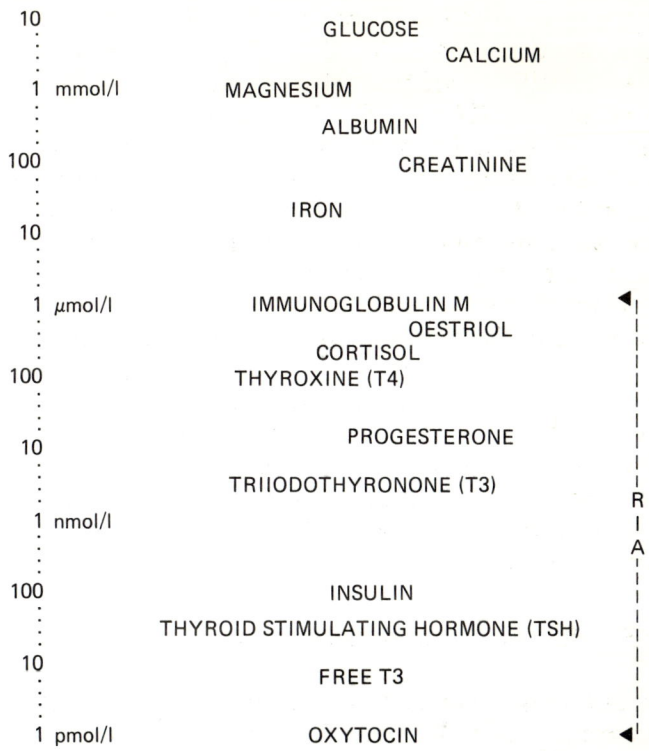

Figure 1.1 *Different substances in human blood at their relative concentrations, with the range of concentrations measured by radioimmunoassay.*

The increase in *sensitivity* can be illustrated by considering Figure 1.1. This figure shows a number of substances of biological significance that are found in blood, ranked in positions indicating their approximate concentrations. At the time of the Berson and Yalow publication the lower limit of detection using established physico-chemical procedures was approximately 10^{-8} to 10^{-9} moles. Study of substances at lower concentrations had to be carried out by experimental inferences and deductions, and where necessary using radioisotopic tracing techniques. As indicated in Figure 1.1, the range of potential detection using RIA considerably extended the list of substances that would be subject to direct quantitation. It opened up new windows on physio-

4 *Immunoassay*

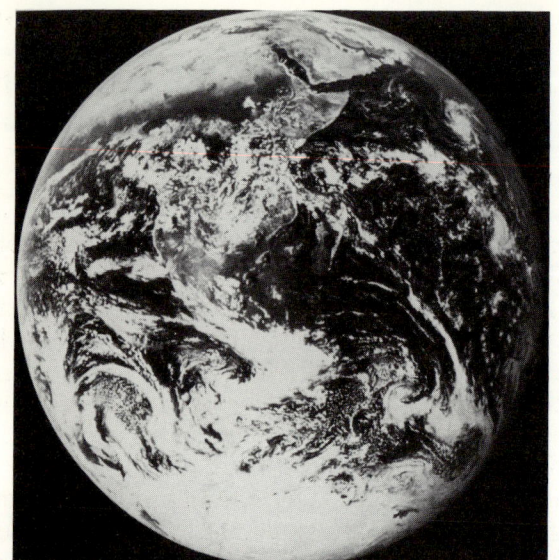

a)

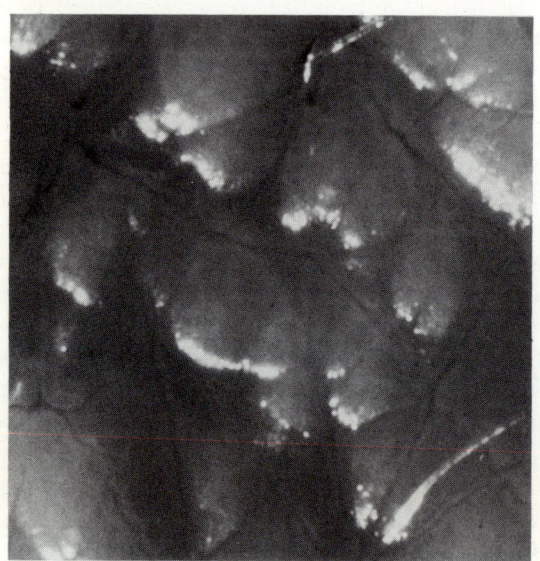

b)

logical processes, which until that time were very difficult to study directly with any accuracy. The full scale of the increase in sensitivity of measurement is perhaps difficult to appreciate from this diagram. For example, the concentration axis in Figure 1.1 is expressed logarithmically and it is undoubtedly difficult to translate the difference in these concentration terms into mental concepts. A suitable, if dramatic, illustration of the difficulty in conceptualising these differences can be appreciated by considering the following example. The difference between the top and bottom concentration in Figure 1.1 is a factor of 1×10^{10} or, a ten thousand million fold difference. If this difference were translated into visual terms, the view of our planet Earth from space (Figure 1.2a), if magnified by this factor (1×10^{10}), would show the details of Figure 1.2b. A magnification of this factor reveals a piece of epidermis (only 1.4 mm across) on the arm of one of the human inhabitants. This illustration may make it easier to appreciate the potential advantage of the RIA in terms of sensitivity when related to other analytical techniques.

The potential *specificity* of RIA is illustrated in Table 1.1. This table shows the potency of various steroids when reacted with an antiserum for the oestrogenic steroid oestradiol-17β. In this example, it is seen that the closely related oestrogenic steroid oestrone has a potency of 0.5%, or only ¹⁄₂₀₀ that of oestradiol-17β. Looking at the molecular structures of these two steroids, shown diagrammatically in Figure 1.3, the small changes of molecular structure, that the RIA is specific for, can be appreciated.

The apparent *simplicity* of RIA, once the reagents were prepared, was of obvious interest. Using these techniques, it seemed possible to investigate small volumes of biological fluids, such as blood or urine directly, i.e. without prior

Figure 1.2 *The difference between 10 mmoles and 1 pmole (or, for example, the difference between the concentration, in blood, of glucose and that of oxytocin, see Figure 1.1). The scale of this difference can be very difficult to appreciate. The illustration given in the two photographs may be useful. (a) At a certain position in space, a view of the Earth shows these details. (b) From the same position, if the field of view were magnified by a factor of 10^{10} (i.e. the difference between 10 mmoles and 1 pmole), it would be possible to see the detail on a piece of human skin just 1.4 mm across.*

Table 1.1
Relative Potency of Steroids with Anti-Oestradiol-17β Serum

Oestradiol-17β	100·0
Oestrone	0·5
Oestradiol-17α	2·0
Oestradiol-17β glucuronide	<0·1
Dihydrotestosterone	0·2
Androst-5-ene 3β-17β-diol	0·1
5α androstane-3β-17β-diol	0·06
Epitestosterone	0·1

work up, like extraction and subsequent purification or concentration. Because manipulations were kept to a minimum, many more samples could be analysed at one time. These advantages of simplicity in an analytical technique were going to increase the speed at which any investigation using these methods could progress.

The other important aspect of RIA was that it was a technique not restricted to a limited group of chemical substances, but capable of almost *universal application*. The term 'universal' is used here to imply a wide variety of different substances. Work in the 1950s had already shown that antisera could be produced to a range of chemical substances and, in particular, it was known that even small molecules, that were not immunogenic in themselves, could stimulate the production of specific antisera when covalently

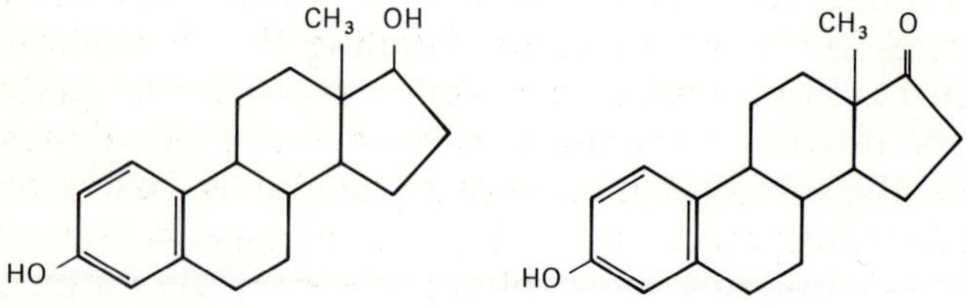

Figure 1.3 *Chemical structures of the two relevant oestrogens listed in Table 1.1, illustrating the discrimination possible with an antibody.*

coupled to larger immunogens like the protein albumin (see p. 58, Chapter 5).

None of these four features were individually unique. In 1944, Landsteiner had clearly demonstrated the potential specificity of antisera when he showed that they could distinguish between stereo-isomeric forms of tartaric acid. Indeed, in 1951 Boydon had published the general principle for an increase in sensitivity when using an early form of an immunoassay and, in 1954, Stavitsky and Arguilla had described an immunoassay method together with many of the relevant parameters. But it was undoubtedly the work of Berson and Yalow that brought together all these features and indicated the true potential of the application. The significance of their work is amply illustrated by the fact that Dr Yalow was to share in the award of a Nobel prize in 1977, an award given primarily for the importance of the application of RIA in the medical field.

Theory of Immunoassay Practice

During the time that Berson and Yalow in the USA were detailing the first radioimmunoassay, an identical assay system (identical in all but name) was proposed by Ekins in England. His use of the term 'saturation analysis' was invoked to indicate the much wider application of a fundamental method, where other specific binding agents could substitute for the antibody.

Although the term 'saturation analysis' was not widely adopted, the work of Ekins detailing the theoretical background to immunoassays has been important in guiding the general development and improvement of techniques.

The theory of immunoassay practice is based on very simple concepts, such as the law of mass action and the Langmuir theory of adsorption; however, the mathematical formulation of specific situations can appear very complex. For this reason, many workers have dispensed with the theoretical predictive approach to rely almost entirely on subjective empirical development. For this reason, the translation by Ekins, and others, of theoretical predictions into practice has been useful.

Alternatives to Radioisotopes

A certain emotive and professed anxiety about the use of radioisotopes, although usually unfounded, (as will be discussed later), may well have led to the widespread search for alternative methods of detection, such as enzyme reactions and fluorophores. The significance of the radioisotopic 'label' was that it undoubtedly led to enhanced sensitivity. However, certain markers, other than radioisotopes, can be successfully used to give specific immunoassays. The publication mentioned earlier of Stavitsky and Arquilla in 1954 described an immunoassay where measurement was by agglutination of red blood cells coupled to the immunological reagent. This technique of monitoring immunological reactions with the aid of red blood cells (see p. 124, Chapter 10) was one of the earliest examples of 'labelled' immunoassay methods. In fact, red blood cells were important in elucidating the much earlier descriptions of haemolysin by Bordet in 1898, and the complement fixation process in 1901 (see p. 131, Chapter 10).

Fluorophores have also been proposed as suitable alternatives to the use of radioisotopic 'labels'. Perhaps the use of the word 'alternative' gives the mistaken impression that the use of fluorophores has been a recent development arising out of the practice of radioimmunoassay. This is not the case, since fluorescent labelled antibodies had been in use for at least two decades prior to the first radioimmunoassay.

Unlabelled Immunoassays

The use of a 'labelled' reagent, be it either radioisotope, red blood cell or fluorophore, obviously enhanced the sensitivity of immunoassay work. However, immunoassay methods with unlabelled reagents had been in use for many years. The reaction between soluble antisera and antigens, giving rise to insoluble precipitates visible to the eye was noted as early as 1897 by Krause. This fundamental aspect of immunoprecipitation was to provide the basis of a quantitative immunoassay method described by Heidelberger and Kendall in 1929 and 1935, and called the precipitin test. This precipitin test (see p. 111, Chapter 9) includes many, if not all, of the characteristics which were to be described much later in the various publications of radioisotopically labelled immunoassay methods.

Of course, there are several immunoprecipitation assay methods which use the formation of a precipitation line and its position in gels for detecting and measuring the extent of reaction between the reagents and analytes. A number of publications from 1945 onwards, from authors like Oudin, Ouchterlony and Laurell, describe the basic aspects of different immunoprecipitation assays in gels. Again, this work is pre-dated by many years by the work of Bechold in 1905. Bechold described the precipitin reaction in gels, but the use of this finding as an analytical tool was not to be considered again until many years later. The fact that Bechold was a physicist and not an immunologist was undoubtedly a significant factor. Segregation within scientific disciplines can be very effective.

The Development of Antisera

Undoubtedly, the full potential of radioimmunoassay, and of immunoassay methods in general, would not have been realised without the many years of development in the study of antibodies. The work in the 1920s recognising an optimal proportion of antibody to antigen required for reaction was obviously important, as it indicated the quantitative nature of the immunological reaction. Considerable work on the nature of antigenic determinant groups of epitopes and the application of the hapten principle (see p. 58, Chapter 5) during the 1930s and the 1940s illustrated both the potential specificity of antibodies and the wide range of molecules against which antibodies could be raised. Subsequent advances in the 1950s on antibody structure and cellular immunity, whilst interesting, have not been very relevant, as yet, to the application of immunoassay methods.

One of the most significant developments in the production of highly specific antisera has been the more judicious use of small amounts of immunogen. Taking one example raising antisera to the pituitary hormone prolactin, it is interesting to note that the original publications on the subject in 1938 detailed the use of 200–300 mg of prolactin in an injection schedule. Today, it is usual to inject approximately 50–100 µg per animal, two or three times a year. Undoubtedly, the excessive amounts of immunogen used originally were detrimental to the production of high affinity and specific antibodies, presumably through induction of immune tolerance.

The Development of a Simple Solid-Phase Reagent

It is often the case that the most simple discovery can have the most widespread effects on subsequent developments. One such innovation has been the property of antibodies, which as proteins, become strongly adsorbed onto plastic surfaces, usually at pH 9–10. In 1967, Catt and Tregear described the adsorption of antibodies onto polystyrene and polypropylene discs. Through the courtesy of the petroleum industry, these plastics can now be found in almost any laboratory and dedicated to almost any use. As a consequence, immunoassays are carried out with reagents stuck to plastic discs, plastic beads, plastic tubes, plastic wells, plastic trays and plastic particles. The fact that these solid-phase reagents can be prepared simply and readily, if not always reproducibly, has done much to both popularise immunoassay methods and vastly increase the sample throughput of quantitative and qualitative techniques. As is the case for many 'innovations', a similar discovery was made earlier, in 1956, when Singer and Plotz described the adsorption of antibodies onto polystyrene latex.

Reagent 'Kits'

In the 1960s various commercial enterprises entered the field with the provision of immunoassay reagents in the form of 'kits'. The involvement of commercial interests, in part, explains the introduction of a very competitive nature in immunoassay development and the consequent proliferation of methodology. It is quite possible that the application of the patent system acted as a considerable stimulus to the subsequent development of alternative approaches.

Perhaps the most significant aspect of the phenomenon of reagent 'kits' is that it indicates both the technical skill necessary for the provision of good quality immunoassay reagents and methods, and the scale of production necessary to ensure consistency in immunoassay performance.

Postscript

This brief historical survey of the development of immunoassay methods is a personal and subjective view of what are felt to be the more significant events. Undoubtedly, other views would highlight different areas and consider other events as significant. The purpose of this review was not to present an objective account of immunoassay evolution, a difficult, if not impossible, task, but simply to introduce certain subjects and to indicate the general interest shown over the years in these techniques.

Further Reading

Ciba Foundation Colloquia on Endocrinology (1962). *Immunoassay of Hormones*, Vol. 14. London: J. & A. Churchill Ltd.

CHAPTER TWO

Basic Concepts in Immunoassay

Introduction

The theory behind immunoassay practice for many workers appears to be too complex, particularly for the non-mathematician. This impression of difficulty is misleading in that the basic principles and concepts of immunoassay methods are quite simple, and an understanding of the basic concepts used is important in both the development and application of different immunoassay methods. Although complex mathematical formulations of immunoassay reactions are useful for identifying relationships between the various components and, thus, to predict optimal procedures, it is not necessary to be fully conversant with these, as successful immunoassay practice can be, and often is, carried out empirically.

Another confusing aspect of immunoassay theory is the apparent contradictory use of terminology. In general, the confusion arises because different authors have used the same term to convey slightly different meanings. Once the basic concepts and definitions are understood, these apparent contradictions are usually resolved.

The Antibody Molecule

The critical component of an immunoassay is an antibody, being a molecule produced *in vivo* (see p. 55, Chapter 5). The antibodies present in antisera are large molecules with molecular weights usually >150 000 daltons. They are proteins belonging to the immunoglobulin (Ig) class. Immunoglobulins are divided into a number of sub-groups, which are indicated by letters; for example, IgG, IgA, IgM, IgD and IgE. Many of the antisera used in immunoassay systems contain antibodies predominantly of the IgG, IgM or possibly IgA subclass.

Most, if not all, antibodies have the basic molecular structure illustrated in Figure 2.1. As indicated in this figure, the binding site for an antigen is located in the variable region. The terms 'constant region' and 'variable region' refer to constancy or variability of the amino acid sequence within a class of immunoglobulins. Variations in amino acid sequence give rise to the variety of different antigen binding sites. So a specific amino acid sequence and, of course, the subsequent tertiary structure of that part of the protein, determine the given specificity of the antigen binding site. It has been calculated that these variations in structure can potentially give rise to 10^{10} different antigen binding sites.

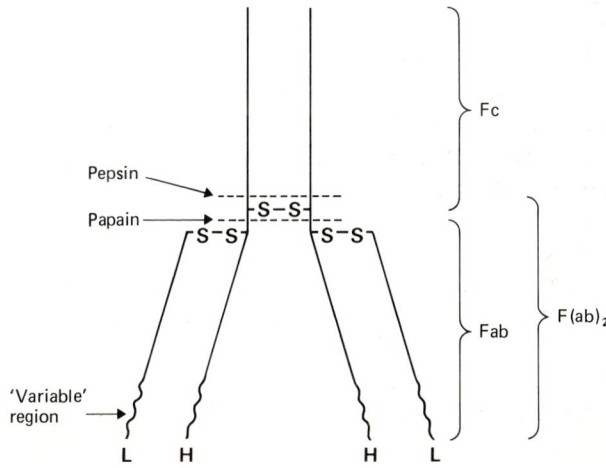

Figure 2.1 *Basic structure of an antibody molecule; the molecule consists of two long or heavy (H) chains and two shorter or light (L) chains. Cleavage by the proteolytic enzymes, pepsin or papain, yields either F(ab)₂ or Fab and Fc fragments. The 'variable' region contains the antigen-binding site.*

The Immunoassay

An immunoassay is essentially the measurement of a substance using the reaction of an antibody, the immunoreagent. The word measurement implies both quality and quantity. At the beginning of the reaction, the antibody (Ab) and the antigen (Ag) associate to form a complex (Ab:Ag), i.e:

$$Ab + Ag \rightarrow Ab{:}Ag$$

This reaction is reversible, and so the complex will dissociate. As more complex is formed there will be an increasing amount of dissociation, i.e:

$$Ab{:}Ag \rightarrow Ab + Ag$$

After a certain time, the net association will be balanced by the same amount of dissociation and the reaction will be at equilibrium, i.e:

$$Ab + Ag \rightleftharpoons Ab{:}Ag$$

The affinity of the antibody for its antigen is a measure of strength of the binding between the antibody and antigen in the complex. The higher the affinity the more antibody and antigen will be complexed at equilibrium. For many antibodies the affinity of the reaction with the antigen is very high.

An assay is simply an attempt to answer the question 'How much of what?'. As was illustrated in Table 1.1, antibodies have the potential for very high specificity, and thus are ideally suitable for defining the 'what' of the question.

In defining the 'how much' of the question, assays using antibodies can be classified in one of two basic procedures. This classification is based on whether the antibody (the specific reagent) is used at a limited concentration, or whether the antibody is used in excess. Based on a common, but not universal, usage these methods can be termed the 'immunoassay', where the antibody is limited, and the 'immunometric assay', where the antibody is in excess. As will be seen later (see p. 111, Chapter 9) there is a third type of immunoassay method where the assay design allows the antibody and antigen to react in approximately equal proportions, so the antibody is neither limited or in excess. The term immunoassay method is used in a generic sense to mean assays of all types.

Immunoassay; a Limited Amount of Reagent

The immunoassay is represented diagrammatically in Figure 2.2. Varying concentrations of antigen are allowed to react with a constant and a limited amount of antibody. The term limited is used to imply that the molar concentration of antibody is much lower than the molar concentration of antigen to be assayed. This aspect of the immunoassay is unusual in that, for most assay methods, the critical reagent is present in excess.

After reacting until there is no further net association or dissociation of antibody and antigen, i.e. at equilibrium, the situation on the right-hand side of the diagram is reached. Given a high affinity between the antibody and the antigen, most, or for purposes of the illustration, all of the antigen binding sites are occupied by antigen, with an increasing concentration of antigen not complexed or not bound to the antibody. These two states of the antigen are commonly

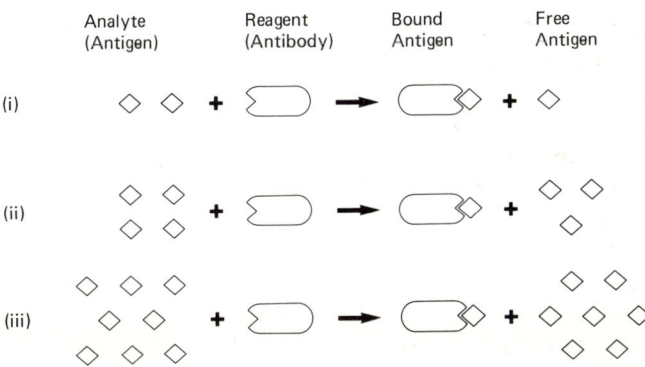

Figure 2.2 *Immunoassay; with a 'limited' concentration of antibody, varying concentrations of antigen give rise to increasing proportions of antigen in the free fractions.*

referred to as bound (to the antibody) and free (not bound) fractions. By measuring the proportion of antigen distributed between the bound and free fractions, one arrives at a relationship where, for example, the amount bound, expressed as a percentage, varies inversely to the concentration of the antigen. This relationship is illustrated in Figure 2.3.

16 Immunoassay

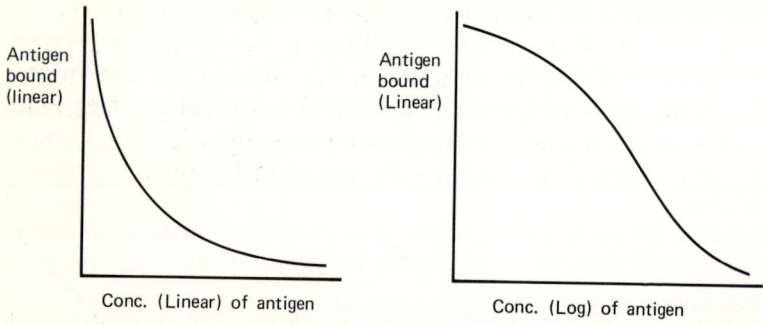

Figure 2.3 *Plots of the relationship between proportion of antigen in the bound fraction and concentration of antigen on a linear and a logarithmic scale.*

Immunometric Assay; Reagent in Excess

The essential aspect of this method is illustrated in Figure 2.4. As before, varying concentrations of antigen are allowed

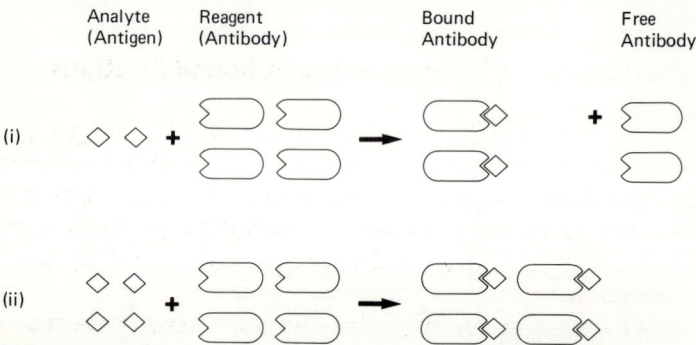

Figure 2.4 *Immunometric assay; with an 'excess' of antibody, increasing concentrations of antigen give rise to a corresponding increase in bound antibody.*

to react with a constant and 'an excess' amount of antibody. 'Excess' is defined as a much higher molar concentration of antibody than the molar concentration of antigen.

After a given time the components will have reacted and reached equilibrium. As before, given a high affinity between antibody and antigen, an increasing proportion of the antibody concentration will have reacted with the antigen, as shown on the right-hand side of Figure 2.4. In the immunometric assay, it is the distribution of antibody between the free and bound fractions that is measured, and not the antigen, as in the immunoassay. The resulting relationship between bound antibody varying directly with the increasing concentration of antigen is given in Figure 2.5.

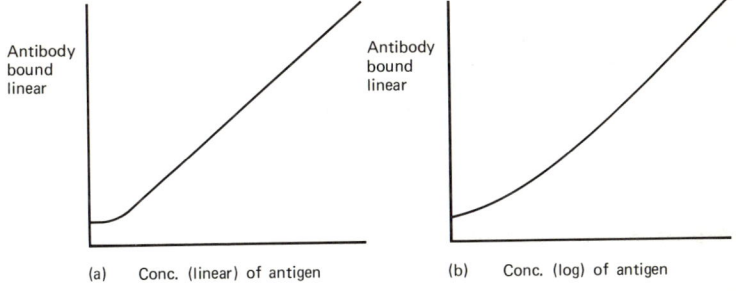

Figure 2.5 *Plots of the relationship between bound antibody and concentrations of antigen on a linear or a logarithmic scale.*

Discrimination between Free and Bound Fractions

In order to monitor the free and bound fractions of either antibody or antigen, it is necessary to be able to discriminate clearly between the two fractions. Discrimination between the two fractions is usually achieved by physical separation of the reaction into two distinct portions: a precipitate, and a supernatant.

Separation usually relies on the distinct nature of the antibody, and where this differs from the nature of the antigen. The antibody is a protein (an immunoglobulin) with a molecular weight usually greater than 150000 daltons. It can be separated from antigens, which are usually much smaller molecules, by a variety of physico-chemical techniques.

The physico-chemical techniques used for separation are given in Table 2.1. Each technique will have its own particular advantages and disadvantages. These are not always predictable and may need empirical evaluation for a particular antibody and antigen reaction.

Table 2.1
Separation

Basis	Method	Feature
Molecular charge	Electrophoresis	Can remove interfering factors including damaged tracer
Molecular size	Chromatography	
	Adsorption	Non-specific adsorption of small molecules, e.g. charcoal
	Diffusion	Usually used in conjunction with other systems, like second antibody
	Filtration	
Proteins	Precipitation of proteins	Using polyethylene glycol (6000) or ethanol. Not very specific
Immunoglobulins	Immuno-precipitation	Second antibody or protein A. Usually quite specific
General	Solid-phase reagent	For example, plastic surfaces, cellulose particles or magnetic beads. Can be very specific

Quantitation

In addition to separating the bound and free fractions, there is a requirement for quantitation of the fractions. The amount of either antigen or antibody in the bound and free fractions can be measured directly. In the quantitative precipitin test (see p. 111, Chapter 9) the nitrogen content of the complexed and precipitated antigen–antibody is measured directly by the micro-Kjeldahl technique. The protein content of the precipitate can also be measured by a specific colour reaction, such as the Folin-Ciocalteau test.

The complex of antigen and antibody can also be measured by a visual precipitation line in gels, for example, immunodiffusion or immuno-electrophoresis assays. In these assays, the free antigen or antibody diffuse or electrophoretically migrate away, and hence are separated from the bound fraction.

The attachment of either antigen or antibody to cells or particles leads to visual agglutination of the cells or particles

Table 2.2
Commonly used 'Labels' in Immunoassay Methods

Nitrogen in precipitate
Visual precipitation line
Red cells
Particles
Scattering of light
Radioisotope
Enzyme
Fluorophore
Luminescence

when the antigen and antibody react together. The use of cells or particles as 'labels' added to antibody or antigen and subsequent visual agglutination improves the sensitivity of detection. The use of other 'labels', e.g. radioisotopes, with much greater detector responsivity, has led to a considerable improvement in the sensitivity of immunoassay methods. 'Labels' linked to antigens or antibodies provide a measurement or detection which can directly relate to the concentration of the particular reactant in a fraction.

'Labels' used for detection and measurement of the free or bound fractions are listed in Table 2.2. The type of label is often the most distinguishing aspect of an assay. Hence, it is the basis of the system of classification, given in Table 2.3,

Table 2.3
A Simple Classification of Immunoassay Methods
(based on detection and relative concentration of reagent)

Detection	Limited reagent	Equivalence	Excess reagent
Nitrogen in precipitate		Precipitin test	
Precipitation line (visual)		Immunodiffusion Immunoelectrophoresis	
Agglutination			Haemagglutination Latex agglutination
Light scattering			Nephelometric Turbidimetric
Radioisotope	Radioimmunoassay (RIA)		Immunoradiometric (IRMA)
Enzyme	Enzymoimmunoassay (EIA)		Enzyme-labelled Immunosorbent (ELISA)
Fluorescence	Fluoroimmunoassay (FIA)		Immunofluorometric (IFMA)
Luminescence	Luminoimmunoassay (LIA)		Immunoluminometric (ILMA)

which used in conjunction with the simple categories already introduced, provides a framework for understanding the principles involved. For example, for a radioisotopic label there is the radioimmunoassay (limited reagent) and immunoradiometric assay (excess reagent).

Characteristics of Antibodies

As has already been noted, RIA literature is beset by a number of terms which, in places, seem to be defined in ways which can only be described as contradictory. It may be useful to realise that some of the common terms either describe aspects of the antibody, or aspects of the assay.

The *titre* is perhaps the first term commonly encountered in immunoassay literature. Titre is a measure of the amount of antiserum needed to complex a given quantity of antigen (see p. 58, Chapter 5, for a fuller description). At this stage it is simpler to consider the antiserum as a fixed concentration of antibody and thus, antiserum is practically synonymous with antibody. The titre of an antiserum may be used to denote the quality of the material, but this is misleading as it is really a quantitative term, which only indicates the amount to be used.

Specificity, in general, describes the uniqueness, or lack of such, of the binding site on an antibody for an antigen. Thus, a highly specific antibody will be understood to possess binding sites which interact only with an antigen with a unique molecular structure. Conversely, a non-specific antibody would react with a variety of antigens showing different molecular structures.

Valency refers to the number of potential binding sites on an antibody for a specific antigen. As antibodies have an essential bilateral structure, the valency of most antibodies is at least two. Thus, many antibodies are bivalent or multivalent (i.e. many binding sites). However, if the antibody is used at a sufficiently low concentration, or as often described in immunoassay terms, high dilution, it may well act as a monovalent component.

The term *avidity* is used to denote the potential antigen binding displayed by an antibody. An antibody with high avidity will display a tendency to bind a lot of antigen and, conversely, an antibody with low avidity will have a tendency to bind few antigen molecules. It is useful to realise that this term does not necessarily describe the strength or affinity of binding, and is not synonymous with affinity. Avidity is obviously a reflection of both the strength of binding, affinity, and the number of binding sites (valency).

Characteristics of Assays

Whereas the terms described above are perhaps best considered as descriptive of the antibody molecule, terms like accuracy, affinity and precision can be seen as a reflection of assay, and not antibody characteristics, although they may be conveying similar concepts.

Accuracy is usually used to denote the ability of an assay system to generate a correct result. As such, it conveys similar concepts to the term specificity but, of course, it also relates to other aspects such as precision. For example, a result can be incorrect because the assay system is sensitive to inappropriate substances, i.e. lack of specificity, or because it is sensitive to small changes, i.e. imprecise.

A useful device to illustrate the concepts involved is the target shown in Figure 2.6. This illustration considers various results of firing a missile at a target, where the aim is to hit the 'bull'. From this illustration it can be appreciated that the accurate method, or that which gives the 'correct' or desired results, is the method that is precise without a bias.

The term *affinity* is used to describe the strength of binding between an antibody and an antigen. Thus high affinity can be seen as binding involving a lot of energy or lasting a long time. As affinity is a measure of binding between the antibody and antigen, strictly speaking it should not be used to describe an antibody. However, it can, and frequently is, used to characterise an antibody where it is accepted or assumed that a constant system and similar antigen is being used.

In immunoassay literature, frequent reference is made to affinity by use of a term called the equilibrium constant or the affinity constant (K). K is a simple quantitative term

22 *Immunoassay*

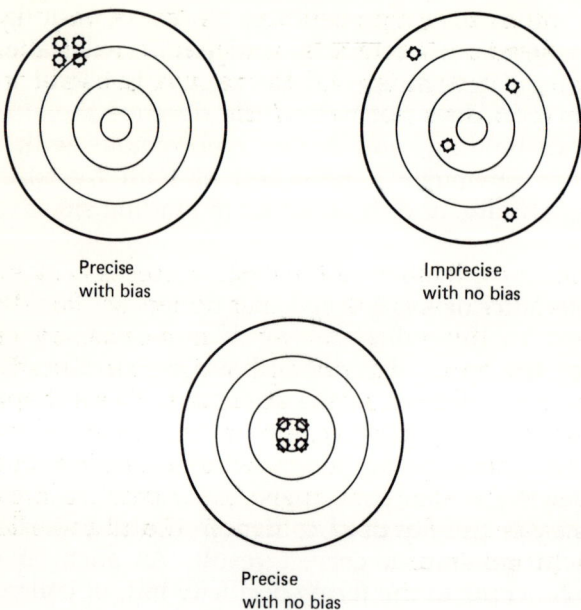

Figure 2.6 *An illustration of the terms 'precise' and 'bias'. Accuracy implies a precise result with no bias.*

described by the following equations:

$$[Ab] + [Ag] \underset{Kd}{\overset{Ka}{\rightleftharpoons}} [Ab:Ag]$$

At equilibrium, the concentrations [ ] of Ab, Ag and Ab:Ag complex will be constant, where Ka is the constant for the rate of association, and Kd is the constant for the rate of dissociation.

$$\text{The equilibrium constant } K = \frac{[Ab:Ag]}{[Ab][Ag]} \text{ or } \frac{Ka}{Kd}$$

or the concentration of complex in molar terms divided by the product of the concentration of the two 'free' components.

For many common immunoassay systems, the equilibrium constant will vary from 1×10^7 litres/mol (low affinity) to

1×10^{11} litres/mol (high affinity). A low affinity system is used to measure substances at higher concentration and a high affinity system is used to measure substances at very low concentrations, e.g. pmol/litre.

Resume

This brief consideration of the basic concepts is by no means exhaustive. However, those mentioned so far should be sufficient for this initial survey of immunoassay methods. Further concepts and principles are introduced, where appropriate, in the subsequent chapters. These chapters deal with the more specific aspects of a variety of methods, classified primarily by the type of detection used. The intention of this survey is to give an understanding of some practical aspects of each type of method and an indication as to its appropriate use.

Further Reading

Kabat E. A. (1980). Basic principles of antigen–antibody reactions. In: *Methods in Enzymology*, Vol. 70: *Immunochemical Techniques, Part A*. London: Academic Press.

Karush F., Otterness I. (1982). Principles of antibody reactions. In: *Antibody as a Tool*. (Marchalonis J. J., Warr G. W., eds.) New York: John Wiley & Sons.

Steward M. W. (1976). *Outline Studies in Biology: Immunochemistry*. New York: John Wiley & Sons.

CHAPTER THREE

Radioimmunoassay

Radioactivity

The significant feature of radioimmunoassay with reference to other immunoassays is the use of a radioisotopic label to discriminate between the antibody bound fraction and the free fraction of the antigen. A radioisotope is essentially an unstable atom which at some time or other will disintegrate and emit sub-atomic particles and/or energy in the form of electromagnetic wave radiation. These particles and/or the energy can then be measured by an appropriate detection system.

The disintegration of any single radioisotopic atom is random, and so it is not possible to predict a time when any given radioisotopic atom will disintegrate. Because radioactive disintegration is a chance event proportional to the

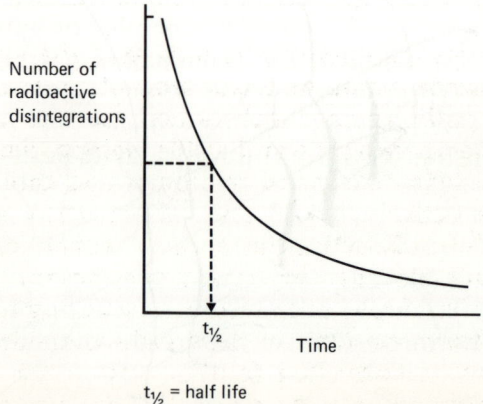

Figure 3.1 *Radioactive decay; the relationship between number of radioactive disintegrations and time. The half life ($t_{\frac{1}{2}}$) is the time for half the number of radioisotopic atoms to disintegrate. Each radioisotope has a distinct $t_{\frac{1}{2}}$.*

total number of radioisotopes present, the number of radioisotopic emissions occurring at one time follows a logarithmic decay curve as shown in Figure 3.1. An important characteristic of this decay is denoted by the half life, i.e. the time taken for radioisotopic atoms to disintegrate leaving half the original number (see Figure 3.1). Each radioactive isotope is characterised by a specific half life, the shorter half lives giving proportionally more disintegrations in a given time.

Different Radioisotopes

The most common radioisotopes used in radioimmunoassays are listed in Table 3.1, together with their characteristic

Table 3.1
Radioisotopes used as Labels in Radioimmunoassay

Radioisotope	Half life	Energy	Detection
^3H	12.26 years β		Liquid scintillation
^{14}C	5730 years β		Liquid scintillation
^{57}Co	270 days γ		Scintillation crystal
^{75}Se	120·4 days γ		Scintillation crystal
^{125}I	60 days γ		Scintillation crystal
^{131}I	8 days $\beta\,\gamma$		Scintillation crystal

half lives, type of energy emitted, and the appropriate detection system. Some radiolabelled antigens can be prepared with radioisotopes substituted for the chemically similar but non-radioactive and stable isotope. For example, the non-radioactive atoms of hydrogen and carbon can be replaced respectively by ^3H and ^{14}C in many molecules. However, the radioactive isotopes of cobalt and iodine would be suitable only in certain specific and particular situations; for example, in the iodine-containing thyronines, the thyroid hormones and in the cobalt-containing vitamin B_{12}. Antigens radiolabelled in this way retain the same chemical configuration as the unlabelled antigen, and invariably exhibit similar binding characteristics to antibodies.

The radioisotopes ^3H and ^{14}C (before detection by liquid scintillation counting) require additional sample preparation

26 *Immunoassay*

and, as a consequence, incur additional expense. Not surprisingly they have been replaced increasingly in popularity by radioisotopes detected by scintillation crystals, and thus, no additional preparation. The most commonly used radioisotope at present is ^{125}I.

Radioiodine Labels

Iodine-125 has many useful attributes as a general radioisotopic label. It is chemically very reactive and can be incorporated into many types of molecules. It is readily available from several commercial sources with virtually 100% radioisotopic purity, i.e. without any non-radioactive iodine. This means that it is possible to incorporate the maximum number of radioactive atoms into a molecule during the labelling process.

The ease of detection is certainly one of the most useful aspects of radioiodine labels. Iodine-125 is detected by

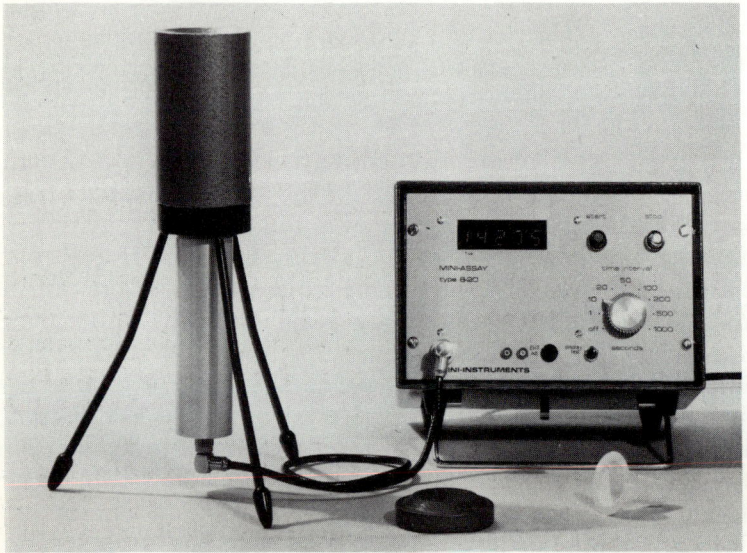

Figure 3.2 *A simple gamma-counter. (Courtesy of Mini-Instruments Ltd, England.)*

placing the sample directly adjacent to a crystal of sodium iodide, containing small amounts of thallium. The gamma-rays from the radioisotope are absorbed by the crystal and the energy is then transmitted in the form of flashes of light. The photons in the crystal are counted by conventional photomultiplier tubes. To increase the efficiency of energy transfer from the isotope to the crystal, a small well is often made in the crystal into which the sample is placed.

There are many references to the high cost of radioisotope detection as a method of quantitation in immunoassay methods. These references are difficult to understand since gamma counters are among the cheapest of all detection instrumentation. A simple gamma counter, for example as shown in Figure 3.2, costs below £500 (1985 price). Compared to the cost of most instrumentation, this represents minimal capital expenditure for a very precise and portable instrument.

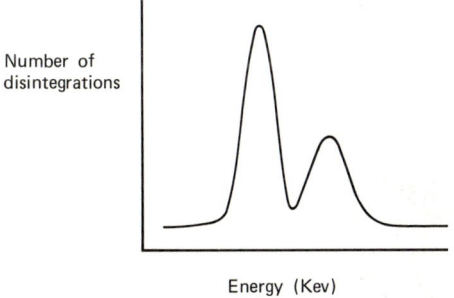

Figure 3.3 *The energy spectrum of ^{125}Iodine; the major peak is at about 27.5 KeV.*

The energy spectrum from ^{125}I (Figure 3.3) is sufficiently high to give efficient detection but not high enough to cause undue concern with regard to radiation hazards. The literature contains many references to the dangers and hazards of radioisotope tracers. These references are not only misleading but, in many cases, grossly inaccurate.

Whilst the handling of mCi amounts of radioiodine during the labelling procedures necessitates care and experience to avoid the hazard of direct ingestion of the volatile radioactive iodine, the use of μCi amounts of label in an assay usually involves the laboratory worker in no real hazard. It is interesting to note that many of the so-called alternative labels may involve much greater hazards; for example, the use of carcinogenic or mutagenic enzyme substrates.

Because radioiodine detection is so simple and efficient, monitoring of contamination is a very easy procedure. Any spillage or contamination with radioiodine can be detected immediately, and appropriate steps taken to remedy the situation. The greatest problem from spillage of radioiodine is not the health hazard but its effect when contaminating the assay, reducing the precision and sensitivity of specific measurements.

Incorporation of Radioactive Iodine – Radioiodination

The basic method for introducing radioiodine into a molecule is by oxidation of sodium ^{125}Iodide to reactive ^{125}I. Iodine will react with the aromatic ring structures of a molecule, resulting in the incorporation of ^{125}I (Figure 3.4).

The usual procedures for oxidising iodide to iodine are given in Table 3.2. The most widely used procedure has been the chloramine T method, published by Hunter and Green-

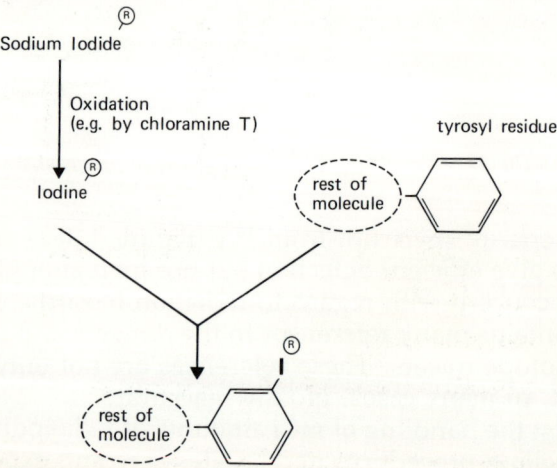

Figure 3.4 *Radioiodination by oxidation of sodium ^{125}Iodide (Ⓡ = radioactive). Iodine can also be incorporated into molecules containing histidine, tryptophan and sulphydryl groups.*

Table 3.2
Methods for Oxidation of Iodide in Radioiodination

Chloramine T	Soluble oxidant
Lactoperoxidase	Enzyme using low concentrations of hydrogen peroxide
Iodogen	Insoluble oxidant

wood in 1962. A milder oxidation reaction can be obtained using the lactoperoxidase enzyme and, if the enzyme is coupled to a solid phase, it can be used very efficiently (Figure 3.5). The solid-phase enzyme is readily removed from the iodination reaction by centrifugation. This can be useful because the enzyme itself will be iodinated and may otherwise be present in the radiolabelled product.

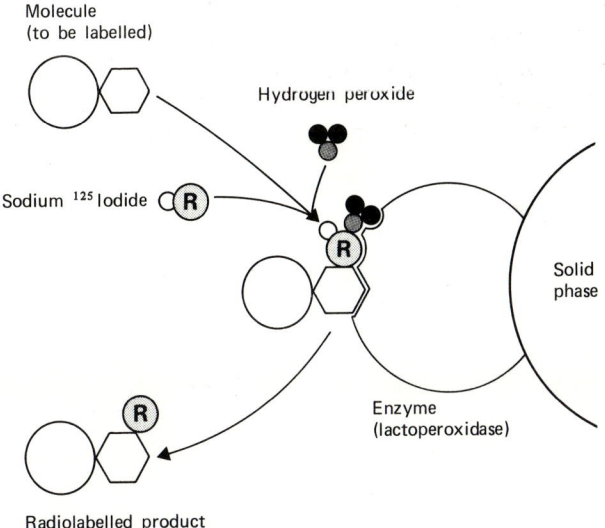

Figure 3.5 *Radioiodination using solid-phase lactoperoxidase.*

Many published methods seem to use far too much oxidant, which will always introduce an additional source of error in the labelling procedure. The excess oxidant can easily oxidise the molecule being labelled, leading to a possible loss of immunological activity. The protocols given in Table 3.3 have been used by the author for many years to radioiodinate a large number and variety of substances with high yields and negligible loss of activity.

Table 3.3
Protocols for Radioiodination

Chloramine T	Solid-phase lactoperoxidase
10 µg Antigen in 10 µl phosphate buffer (pH 7·4, 0·05M)	
10 µl phosphate buffer pH 7·4 (0·5M)	
1mCi ^{125}I(sodium iodide)	
10 µl Chloramine T (10 µg)	10 µl solid-phase lactoperoxidase (approx 10–20 ng enzyme)
	5 µl H_2O_2 (0·5 nmole)
30 seconds	10 minutes
	5 µl H_2O_2 (0·5 nmole)
	20 minutes
10 µl Sodium metabisulphite (10 µg)	100 µl 0·1% azide
100 µl KI (1mg + 1% albumin)	
Purification of products	

Providing the radioactive iodine incorporated into the molecule does not inhibit the antigenic binding function of the antibody, these methods of radioiodination can be used successfully to produce radiolabelled tracers.

Because of the relatively large size of the iodine atom, radioiodination will only be successful in the above terms when the radioiodine is incorporated into a part of the molecule distinct from the antigenic binding site, or when it replaces an endogenous iodine atom as part of the antigenic binding site. In addition, radioiodination will only be useful where the molecule contains constituents which can be substituted with iodine, e.g. tyrosine, histidine, tryptophan or sulphydryl groups. If suitable constituents are missing, or where the substitution of iodine interferes with the antigen-binding function of the antibody, then alternative procedures must be adopted.

Radiolabelling by Conjugation Method

Conjugation labelling has been evolved as a useful method for circumventing the difficulties mentioned above. Essentially, the radioiodine is incorporated into small molecules, such as tyrosine, which can then be coupled to specific sites on the antigen. In these procedures, radioiodination is usually carried out using the chloramine T method, and the resulting radiolabelled substituent is chemically activated prior to coupling with the antigen. This means that the antigen is not subject to the potentially damaging effects of oxidation. One of the most convenient methods of conjugation labelling is with the 'Bolton and Hunter' reagent, named after its originators. The reagent already radioiodinated and purified is available commercially. The 'Bolton and Hunter' reagent is a radioiodinated-active ester which under the appropriate conditions will react with primary amino groups found in peptides or proteins (see Figure 3.6). In some instances, suitably derived analogues are made, introducing an amino group at a specific position in a molecule where none existed previously. In the case of small molecules, this can be arranged to be at a position away from the antigenic binding site, and thus eliminate any interference with the binding of the antibody.

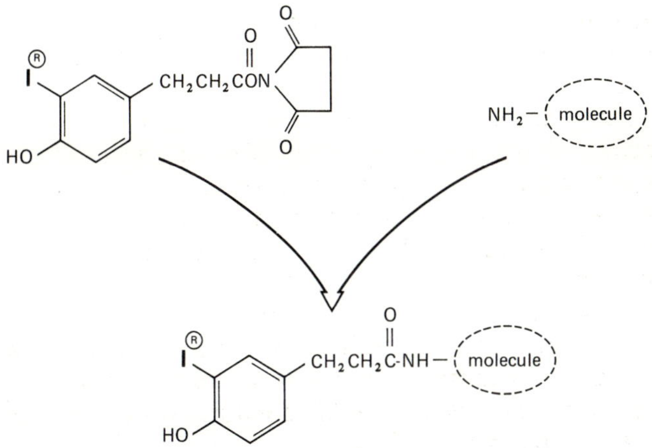

Figure 3.6 *Conjugation labelling. A radioiodinated active ester is reacted with the material to be labelled. The product is a radioactive conjugate.*

Because of the technical complexity of conjugation labelling, it is only considered in those cases where direct radioiodination is not possible, or where it can be shown that direct radioiodination causes a reduction in immunoreactivity.

Purification of Radioiodinated Labels

Irrespective of the method of radiolabelling, the prepared product will require purification before use in radioimmunoassays. To retain the enhanced sensitivity and precision of radioimmunoassays, the purity of the label needs to be high. For most purposes, a satisfactory purity is obtained when chromatographic homogeneity is established. For this reason, the labelled product is immediately separated from impurities by chromatography. The radiochromatographic profile of a typical radioiodination product, as shown in Figure 3.7, illustrates a number of salient points.

In the example given, there are several impurities resolved from the radiolabel other than excess radioiodide. These various constituents often represent material with a higher

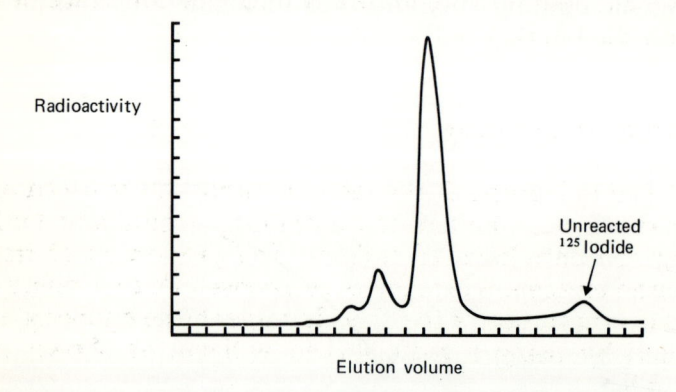

Figure 3.7 *Purification of radioiodination products. In this example, the products from a radioiodination of human prolactin, using solid-phase lactoperoxidase, are chromatographed on Sephadex G100, Superfine (60 × 1 cm). The column is eluted with phosphate buffer (pH 7.4; 0.05M) containing 1% bovine serum albumin and 0.1% sodium azide, at 3 ml/hour. The large monomer peak is separated from small amounts of polymerised (dimer) or aggregated material which display relatively high non-specific binding.*

molecular weight than the radiolabel and may result from polymerisation induced by the oxidation radioiodination process. In some cases they may represent impurities already present in the material to be labelled. In either instance, the presence of these radiolabelled impurities can considerably affect the specificity and precision of the assay. These impurities are often not sufficiently resolved from the labelled antigen when using the common small 'desalting' chromatographic columns.

The use of small 'desalting' columns presupposes that the only impurity is radioiodide. The example given in Figure 3.7 shows that this is patently not the case. Another misleading assumption is that desalting techniques are adequate in separating the small iodide molecule from much larger molecules. Non-specific adsorption of iodide by larger molecules often means that complete resolution of a specific radiolabelled antigen is only possible by extensive chromatography. The resolution can be considerably improved by the presence of sufficient carrier protein in the eluting buffer. The presence of either radioiodide or radiolabelled impurities may give rise to increased blank or background readings in the radioimmunoassay. This, in turn, would lead to a deterioration in the performance of a radioimmunoassay.

The Radioimmunoassay

As detailed in Figure 2.2, the radioimmunoassay is based on the reaction of a limited concentration of antibody with varying concentrations of antigen. The proportion of free and bound antigen, which arises as a consequence of using a limited concentration of the specific reagent (the antibody) is measured by using a radiolabelled antigen, as shown in Figure 3.8.

Radioimmunoassays can use all types of separation techniques (see Table 2.1). The non-specific separations of the antibody fraction (e.g. protein precipitation with ethanol), or non-specific separations of the antigen fraction (e.g. adsorption with charcoal), are being increasingly superseded by specific precipitation methods. The two most specific methods in use are immunoprecipitation, using a second antibody reaction, and separation using solid-phase reagents.

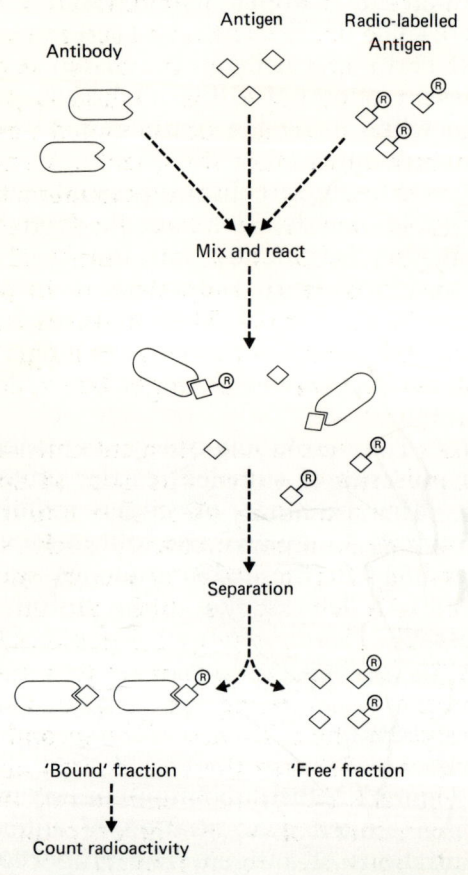

Figure 3.8 *The essential components of a radioimmunoassay.*

Immunoprecipitation with Second Antibody

The second antibody method for immunoprecipitation of the antibody bound fraction has been extensively used for many years. The method requires the use of an anti-Ig serum which reacts with the Ig species of the primary antibody. The primary antibody reacts with the antigen. If the primary antiserum was raised in a rabbit, then the primary antibody would be designated as a rabbit immunoglobulin. In this case, the second antibody would derive from another species of animal (e.g. a donkey) immunised with rabbit immunoglobulins. The donkey antirabbit serum would react specifically with the rabbit primary antibody, leading to a precipitable complex. Although this method is potentially very specific, there are a number of associated non-specific side reactions which can reduce the quality. Many second antibodies will cross-react with immunoglobulins from several species, as those workers who have inadvertently used the wrong type of second antibody can testify. The second antibody may well cross-react completely, or in part, with immunoglobulins in the sample. This produces misleading results where there are high levels of immunoglobulins or immune complexes in samples, as might be expected with rheumatoid conditions.

The precipitable complex is a multivalent complex resulting from the combination of first and second antibodies, each with at least two binding sites. The multimolecular complex can also contain other molecules, such as complement factors, and is often affected by factors such as the concentration of divalent cations, like calcium or magnesium. The use of polyethylene glycol (molecular weight 6000) solutions, usually 4%, to precipitate first and second antibody complexes comprising of just two or three molecules can improve the efficiency of the second antibody precipitation reaction. Because the complexes only involve direct reaction between the primary and second antibodies before precipitation takes place, the non-specific reactions and effects are eliminated or greatly reduced. Not only does this mean that the separation method is more specific but, in addition, it is quicker. It takes much longer to build up large multimolecular complexes than simple bi- or trimolecular complexes.

Separation with Solid-Phase Reagents

Linking antibodies to particles or surfaces gives a solid-phase reagent which can be readily separated from all other components in an immunoassay reaction. Antibodies can be covalently coupled to many different types of particles, such as cellulose, polyacrylamide, polymerised dextrans and nylon. Antibodies can also be strongly adsorbed onto plastic surfaces, such as polystyrene or polypropylene beads and tubes. In all cases, the ease of removing the solid-phase reagent from the reaction mixture greatly enhances the potential specificity of the separation method. In many situations, this potential enhancement is not realised, due to non-specific adsorption reactions of the radiolabel with the vastly increased surface area of the particles. However, because the removal of the solid phase is so readily achieved, this problem can be completely or partially resolved by repeated washing steps. Assays employing solid-phase reagents, together with several washing steps, begin to display the full potential predicted for good radioimmunoassay techniques.

Another important factor in the satisfactory behaviour of particulate solid-phase reagents is the selection of appropriate sized particles. Optimal performance usually results from the use of very small particles (below 10 µm diameter), with a uniform size. One of the difficulties with particulate solid-phase materials is that the particles often have a high density. Depending on the density, they will settle out from the reaction quite rapidly (in minutes rather than hours). If the reaction is proceeding slowly, it is necessary to agitate the tubes to keep the particles in suspension, at least until the reaction nears equilibrium.

The use of solid-phase second antibody resolves some of the difficulties inherent in either the second antibody methods or the solid-phase systems. The reaction between the primary antibody and the antigen proceeds in the liquid-phase and then solid-phase second antibody can be added to precipitate the antibody fraction. If the solid-phase second antibody is added in excess the reaction proceeds quickly, eliminating the need to resuspend the solid-phase. The specificity of this method can be significantly enhanced if purified or epitope-specific second antibodies are coupled to the solid-phase. As solid-phase second antibodies are readily available from several commercial sources (for example, the 'Sac-cel' from Wellcome Diagnostics), this method can be expected to be used extensively.

Salient Features of Radioimmunoassay

The feature most significant in the performance of radioimmunoassay and undoubtedly responsible for the successful application of the technique to measurements in complex biological material is negligible background. Unlike many other labels, the background measurement for radioisotopes like ^{125}I in almost all biological samples is virtually zero. This means that the full sensitivity of radioisotopic detection can be realised. Also, radioactive distintegration is unaffected by changes in physico-chemical parameters such as pH, concentration, temperature, etc. This means that the full specificity of radioisotopic detection can be realised. A few of the alternative labels may offer superior detection characteristics for simple or purified media. However, many of the components of complex biological samples will interfere in the measurement of enzyme reactions, fluorescence, chemiluminescence or any of the other labels.

The hazards or harmful effects of using radiolabelled material are often grossly misrepresented. Quite often the toxicity of these radioisotopes is much less than the toxicity of the carcinogenic or mutagenic materials used in other systems. Although the toxicity of these radioisotopes is negligible in most well ordered laboratories, the strict regulations regarding their use may well occasion some inconvenience. The difficulties encountered will vary considerably throughout the world, but the ubiquitous nature of radioimmunoassay is witness to the satisfactory resolution of these difficulties.

Those isotopes with a relatively short half life, such as ^{125}I, do incur one very significant disadvantage. The practical shelf life of the label is limited to a few weeks or in a few instances to a few months. No matter how stable the radiolabelled material can be made, a fresh preparation will be required when the radioactive disintegration rate falls to such a level that the count rate is too low for practical counting time. In practice, this means that most ^{125}I labelled antigens are prepared every 4–8 weeks. Some ^{125}I labelled antigens, such as steroids, are stable for up to 6 months. However, at the end of that period the counting time would have to be extended by a factor of 8, i.e. three half lives, or $2 \times 2 \times 2$.

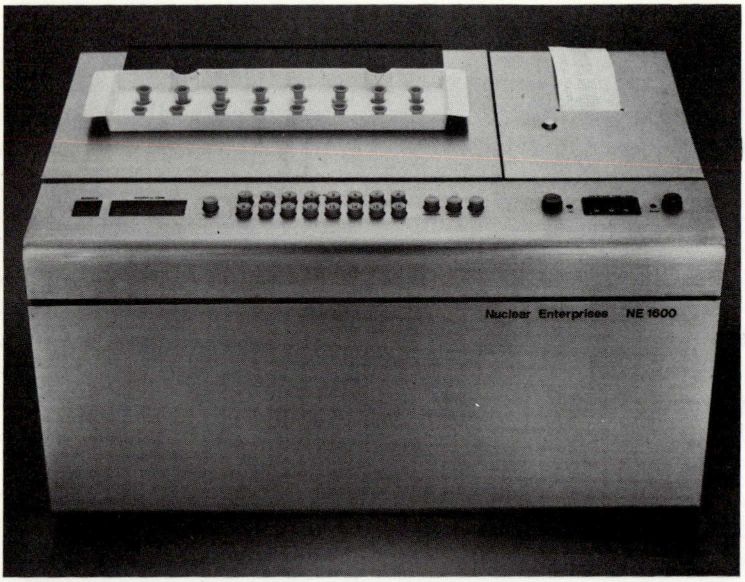

38 *Immunoassay*

Figure 3.9 *A multi-well gamma-counter; this model has 16 wells. Sample throughput with this instrument is equivalent to that from approximately eight conventional automatic gamma-counters, each one costing more than the multi-well counter. (By courtesy of Nuclear Enterprises Ltd, UK.)*

The introduction of multi-well counters (Figure 3.9) for the detection of low energy gamma-rays has been a major advance in the practice of radioimmunoassay. These counters have up to 20 wells and, thus, can process a number of samples at any one time. Because the instruments are dedicated for a fixed and limited range of radioisotopes and are operated manually, they are usually much cheaper than the more flexible and sophisticated automatic gamma-counters.

The potentially limiting parameter in most radioimmunoassays is the separation step. Techniques for the production of pure and stable radiolabelled antigens are now available and in regular use. As a consequence, one of the most common causes of poor performance in radioimmunoassays in the past, that of a 'poor' radiolabel, should have been eliminated or at least dramatically reduced. High affinity and specific antisera can usually be prepared for most antigens. Where this has not been possible, affinity purification or monoclonal production of the required antibodies (see Chapter 5) should prove feasible. Given a satisfactory radiolabel and a satisfactory antisera or antibody, the degree of discrimination between the bound and free fraction becomes the next most important factor. The discrimination between the bound and the free fractions in radioimmunoassays relates to the specificity of the separation method. Commensurate with the need to increase the sensitivity or enhance the specificity of radioimmunoassays, is a requirement to improve the discrimination of the separation methods. It is highly significant that the practice of radioimmunoassays has involved such a wide range of different separation methods, and that the most specific of these are gaining in popularity. The introduction of specifically oriented second antibodies (Chapter 11, p. 154), in conjunction with solid-phase materials, particularly those with low non-specific adsorptive properties, will undoubtedly extend the practical applications of the ubiquitous radioimmunoassay.

Further Reading

Bolton A. E. (1977). *Radioiodination Techniques*. Review 18. Amersham, England: The Radiochemical Centre.

British Medical Bulletin (1974). *Radioimmunoassay and Saturation Analysis*. Vol. 30, No. 1 (entire issue devoted to this subject).

Chard T. (1978). *An Introduction to Radioimmunoassay and Related Techniques*. Amsterdam: Elsevier/North Holland Biomedical Press.

CHAPTER FOUR

Immunoradiometric Assay

Introduction

The radiolabelled antibody immunometric assays or immunoradiometric assays (IRMA) are currently enjoying increasing popularity, and many methods are being developed with a view to replace some of the existing radioimmunoassays. The method was originally published by Miles and Hales in 1968 and, although the potential attributes of the IRMA were strikingly obvious, it is surprising that more use was not made of the method at the time. The current interest is something of a revival, arising perhaps out of the greater availability of purified antibodies (see Chapter 5). Reagent preparation for the immunoradiometric method is often technically more demanding than reagent preparation for the radioimmunoassay. However, the assay is often easier to perform and the IRMA is frequently more precise and has greater sensitivity than the RIA. The IRMA may also have enhanced specificity. These potential advantages are dependent, of course, on the use of reagents and procedures of appropriate quality. In common with RIA the immunoradiometric assay uses radioisotopes and detection of the subsequent radioactivity to measure the antigen concentration. Although theoretically IRMAs could use any one of the radioisotopes used in RIAs, in practice ^{125}I has been used almost exclusively.

Basic Technique

Immunoradiometric assays almost invariably use solid-phase separation techniques to distinguish between the complexed or bound antibody and the unreacted or free antibody. There are a number of general ways in which IRMAs may be performed.

The amount of antigen is measured by the binding of a radiolabelled antibody. Consequently, as the concentration of antigen increases, so does the amount of complexed radiolabelled antibody. This is a direct relationship and, as shown previously (Figure 2.5), is described by the curve repeated in Figure 4.1. The basic immunometric procedure is

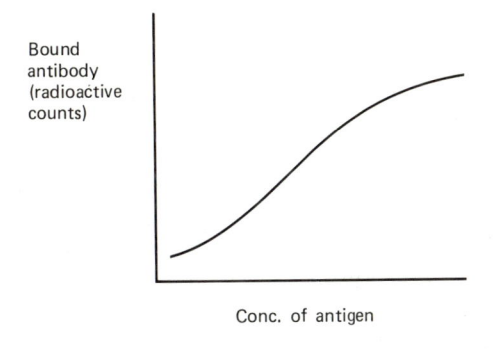

Figure 4.1 *Relationship between bound radiolabelled antibody and concentration of antigen in the immunoradiometric assay.*

shown in Figure 4.2. A solid-phase antigen preparation, again in excess, is added to the reaction tube, where it can bind the 'excess' radiolabelled antibody, or that which has not already reacted, with antigen to be measured. The solid-phase is precipitated, usually by centrifugation, leaving the radioactivity in the supernatant as a direct measure of the concentration of antigen.

'Two-Site' Method

IRMAs may also be performed by the 'two-site' immunometric method. This procedure is illustrated in Figure 4.3. In the two-site immunometric assay the complex of radiolabelled antibody and antigen is precipitated from the reaction mixture by the addition of a solid-phase antibody directed towards the second antigenic binding site on the antigen.

Because of the requirement for two binding sites this refinement is termed the two-site IRMA.

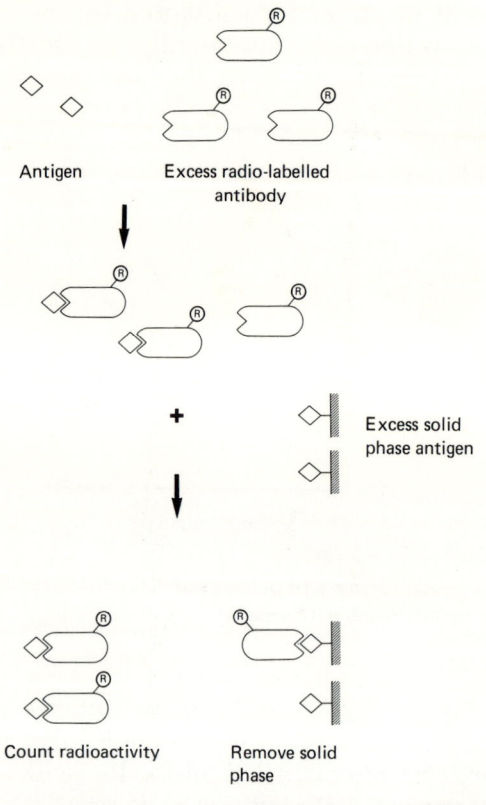

Figure 4.2 *Immunoradiometric assay technique using solid-phase antigen to separate excess radiolabelled antibody from the bound radiolabelled antibody.*

Indirect Labelling

A further modification to the basic IRMA principle was the introduction of indirect labelling of the antibody. Indirect labelling is achieved by using a radiolabelled second antibody, i.e. a radiolabelled antibody for which the antigenic binding site is a portion of the primary antibody. An example of indirect labelling is illustrated in Figure 4.4. Here, the primary antibody itself acts as the antigen for the second

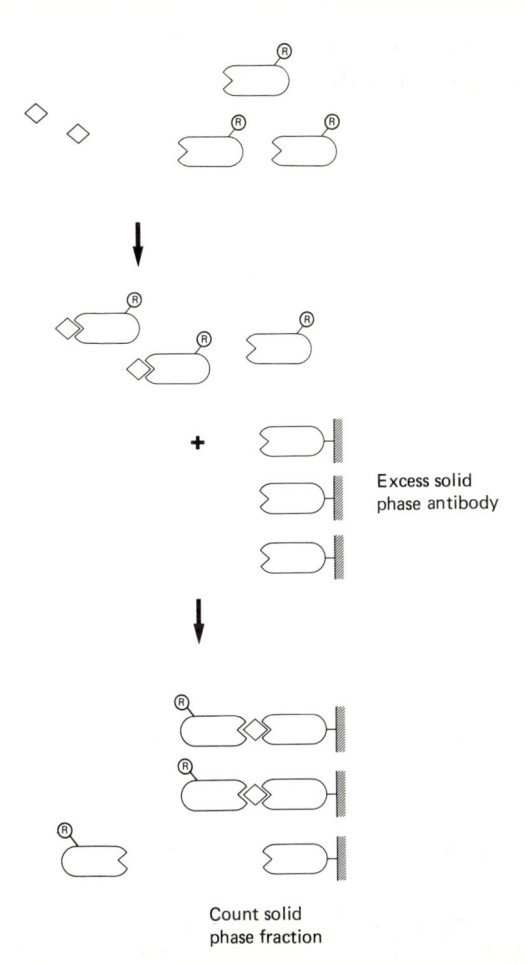

Figure 4.3 *'Two-site' immunoradiometric assay technique; the antigen is bound by two antibodies, therefore two binding sites on the antigen are involved. This technique is also referred to as a 'sandwich' assay.*

antibody. In this case, the second antibody was raised against sheep immunoglobulins and would react with any sheep immunoglobulin of which the first antibody is one.

The pertinent feature of indirect labelling is that it becomes possible to have IRMAs for many different and various antigens and yet use only one type of radiolabelled second antibody. This reduces the complexity of the technical procedures involved in reagent preparation considerably. Although indirect labelling can simplify proceedings, there may be a commensurate reduction in the general performance of the IRMA due to side reactions of a relatively non-specific second antibody.

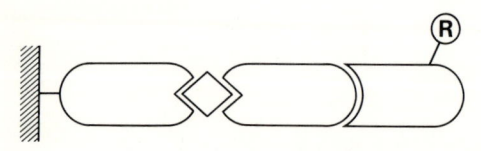

Radio-labelled anti-IgG
(2nd Antibody)

Figure 4.4 *Indirect labelling in an immunoradiometric assay. A radiolabelled second antibody is used to label the primary antibody. The antibody on the solid phase comes from a different animal species to the other primary antibody to avoid labelling any unoccupied solid-phase antibody.*

Sequential Addition of Reagents

For optimal use in IRMAs, different reagents are often added sequentially, allowing time for each reagent to react and then removing the excess before the addition of the next reagent. The presence of a solid-phase with easy precipitation makes the sequential additions technically very simple. The advantage of reacting separate reagents sequentially is found in a reduction of side reactions with the commensurate enhancement of potential sensitivity and specificity. If it is desirable to add all reagents simultaneously it is important to employ only highly purified reagents with specificity for a single antigenic site, or reduce interference by selecting particular concentrations of reagents. For example, in Figure 4.5, where all reagents are added simultaneously, an excess of radiolabelled antibody may interfere with the binding of the solid-phase antibody, (a) if the radiolabelled antibody preparation is a heterogeneous mixture of antibodies to different antigenic sites, or (b) if the antigen has a bilateral distribution of the same antigenic sites. In both situations it is usually possible to eliminate the interference by carefully reducing the concentration of radiolabelled antibody to a critical amount. Of course, any reduction in concentration of the reagents will result in a lengthening of reaction time. By starting with the solid-phase and adding reagents in sequence, very high concentrations may be used with a commensurate decrease in reaction time.

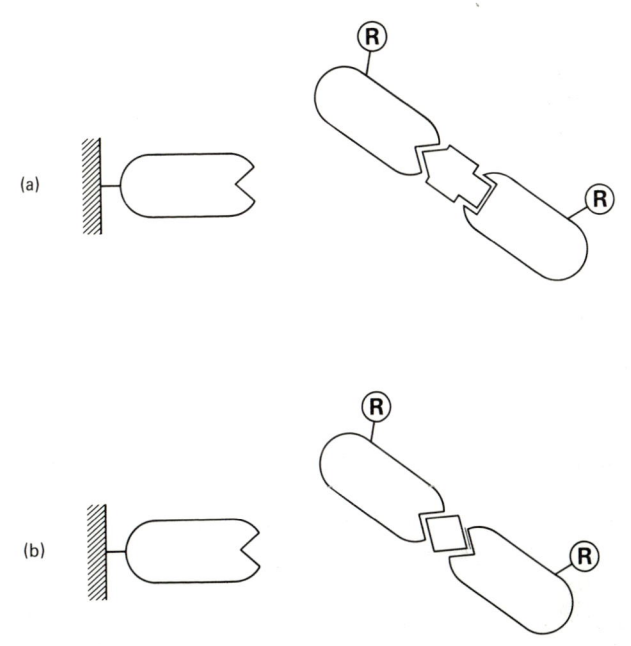

Figure 4.5 *Simultaneous addition of reagent and high concentrations of radiolabelled antibody may inhibit the binding of antigen by the solid-phase antibody, and thus give misleading results. This occurs with (a) a heterogeneous mixture of radiolabelled antibodies, or (b) bivalent antigens.*

Purification of Antibodies

It is necessary to purify antibodies for the preparation of many immunoradiometric reagents. A schematic purification of antibody is given in Figure 4.6, and is discussed at greater length in Chapter 5. Purified antibodies are used in the preparation of radiolabelled antibodies and may be used in the preparation of solid-phase antibodies.

A partially purified preparation (e.g. an IgG fraction of the antiserum) may well be satisfactory for use as a reagent in some IRMAs, particularly where good specificity and high sensitivity are not required. A relevant factor here will be the relative proportion of active antibodies in the immunoglobulin population of the antiserum. If IgG fractions contain predominantly relevant antibodies, further purification may not be necessary.

ANTISERUM
↓ precipitation with ammonium sulphate or sodium sulphate or DEAE ion exchange

IgG FRACTION
↓ react with solid phase antigen (ie. immunoadsorbent)

IMMUNOADSORBED ANTIBODIES
↓ elute immunosorbent pH gradient and other dissociating conditions

SPECIFIC ANTIBODIES

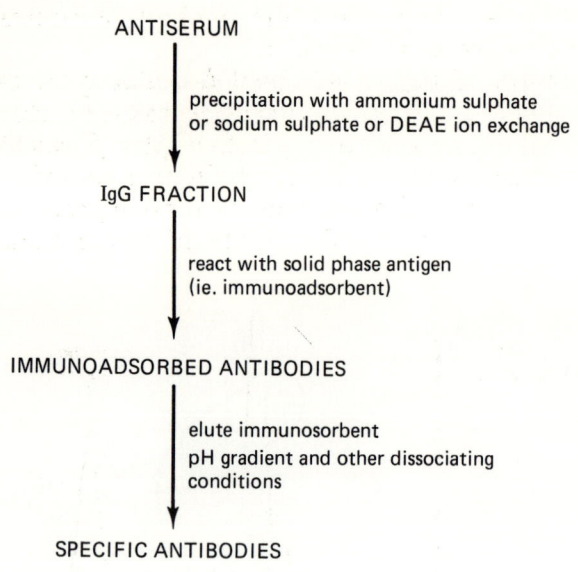

Figure 4.6 *Purification of antibodies from serum.*

Radiolabelling of Antibodies

The radiolabelled antibody is prepared by radioiodination of the purified antibody in an analogous way to the radioiodination of antigens. A summary of the radioiodination techniques used to prepare radiolabelled antibodies is given in Table 4.1. In theory, a different radioiodination technique will be optimal for any one specific antibody preparation. However, because antibodies are chemically very similar, in that they all possess the immunoglobulin protein structure, one method is often practically suitable for all antibody preparations. Chloramine T- or lactoperoxidase-mediated radioiodinations would be the most useful first choices, with

Table 4.1
Methods to Prepare Radiolabelled Antibodies

Chloramine T (soluble oxidant)
Lactoperoxidase (enzymatic oxidation)
Iodogen (insoluble oxidant)
Conjugation labelling (e.g. Bolton and Hunter reagent)

conjugation labelling being the method of choice where stability appears to be a problem.
Purification of the radioiodinated antibody is essential. This is usually achieved by molecular exclusion chromatography. Figure 4.7 shows a chromatographic purification of a radioiodinated sheep antibody. As with radioiodination, a satisfactory purification step suitable for one preparation will often be practical for all other antibody preparations.

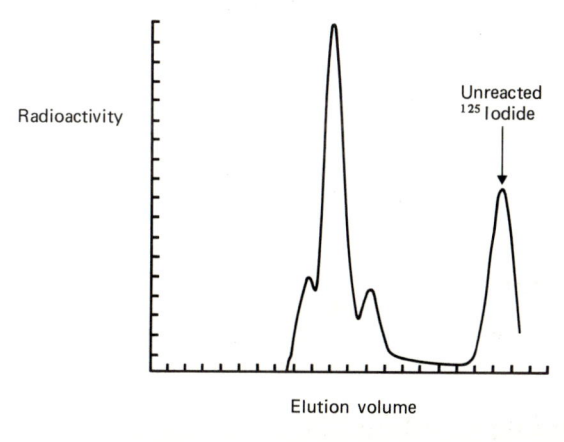

Figure 4.7 *Purification of radioiodinated antibody, a sheep antihuman luteinising hormone, on Sephadex G200, Superfine (45 × 1 cm). The column was eluted with phosphate buffer (pH 7.4; 0.05M), containing 1% bovine serum albumin, 0.1% normal sheep serum and 0.1% sodium azide, at 2 ml/hour. Immunoreactive material, separated from the main peak, gave relatively high non-specific binding (blanks).*

Radioallergosorbent Test (RAST)

A particular example of the immunoradiometric technique is found in the radioallergosorbent test (RAST). This application of the immunoradiometric assay technique measures allergen-specific IgE molecules. It is useful to specify the RAST as it is often classified in the literature as a distinct method. It is also a good example of the practicality of the technique where the antigen is ill-defined or unavailable in the purified state.

Essentially, the test follows the basic pattern of the immunoradiometric method and is outlined in Figure 4.8. A particular allergen, such as pollen or an animal epithelial particle, is coupled to a solid-phase. In some examples of the test, the solid-phase is provided by small discs of paper, giving rise to the acronym PRIST, or paper radioimmunosorbent test! The solid-phase is reacted with the sample containing IgE molecules. The IgE molecules specific to this particular allergen will bind to the solid-phase allergen, and are measured by a radiolabelled anti-IgE antibody. This variation of the immunoradiometric assay is usually semi-quantitative. The allergens are invariably poorly characterised in molecular terms, and there may well be batch-to-batch variation in preparations of allergens. In addition, the allergenic components could well be heterogeneous and not a single entity. This application enables reasonably specific measurements to be made without the need to purify and radiolabel either the allergenic factor or the various anti-IgE antibodies. A single radiolabelled anti-IgE antibody preparation, often directed towards the Fc fragment of the IgE, is sufficient for the measurement, albeit semi-quantitative, of a wide variety of allergens.

The radioallergosorbent test can also be used as a measure of the allergen. The reaction of a preparation of IgE mole-

Solid phase allergen   Radiolabelled anti - IgE

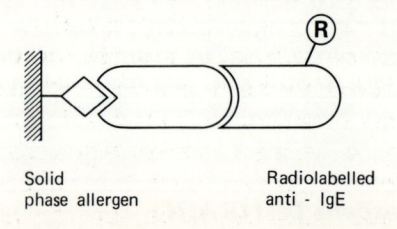

Figure 4.8 *The radioallergosobent test (RAST). A radiolabelled anti-IgE antibody is used to detect specific anti-allergen IgE antibodies absorbed on solid-phase allergen.*

cules with the specific allergen is reduced by the presence of increasing concentration of allergen in the sample (see Figure 4.9). The amount of specific IgE reacted with the solid-phase allergen will be indirectly proportional to the concentration of allergen in the sample. The solid-phase allergen-reacted IgE is then quantified by a subsequent reaction with the radiolabelled anti(Fc)-IgE.

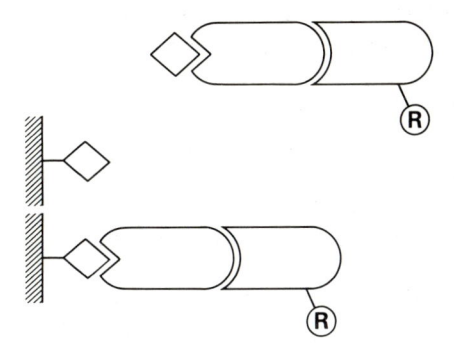

Figure 4.9 *Use of the RAST technique to measure allergens. Allergens in the sample inhibit binding of the specific anti-allergen IgE antibodies to solid-phase allergen. An increasing concentration of allergen would result in a decreasing amount of solid-phase bound radioactivity.*

Salient Features of the IRMA

Where the antiserum has been used for both RIA and IRMA, the IRMA method will often give greater specificity and sensitivity. One important factor in this improvement is the purification of the reagent. It is usual in RIA to use the antiserum with no subsequent purification of the antibody, whereas a purified antibody is invariably used in the IRMA. Both the affinity constant (K value) of the purified antibody and specificity, in terms of percentage cross-reactions, may be considerably improved over the values for the native antiserum (Table 4.2). A value for the native antiserum obviously represents the mean value resulting from the mixture of different populations of antibodies. This average value is often much lower than the optimal figure because it

Table 4.2

	Native antiserum	Purified antibody
K Value, e.g. anti-TSH	2.6×10^{10}	5.2×10^{10}
Cross-reaction, e.g. HPL with anti-GH	0.08%	<0.01%

includes the effect of many low affinity antibodies with reduced specificities.

The improvement in specificity of the purified antibody over the performance of the native antiserum considerably enhances the potential accuracy of immunometric measurements. This important parameter of immunoassay methods has frequently been neglected, usually arising from an excessively dogmatic belief in the specific nature of antibodies.

Precision Profile of Immunoradiometric Assays

One strikingly obvious advantage of the immunoradiometric assay over the radioimmunoassay is the increase in precision as shown by precision profiles. A precision profile is simply a measure of precision in terms of the concentration of analyte, e.g. coefficient of variation for a given concentration plotted against the relevant concentration. Because precision profiles use variations in concentrations (i.e. the result) and not variations of the measurement or response parameter, comparison between the profiles from different methods are usually relevant and valid. If precision profiles for cognate radioimmunoassays and immunoradiometric assays are compared, as in Figure 4.10, the precision of the immunoradiometric assay is invariably better. This improved precision gives the IRMA the characteristics of better sensitivity and a higher detection limit at high concentrations, giving overall a much wider working range. In radioimmunoassays with a limited working range, samples that give results above the upper limit of the range may require reanalysis at a greater dilution. The more extensive range of the immunoradiometric assay allows for direct analysis of

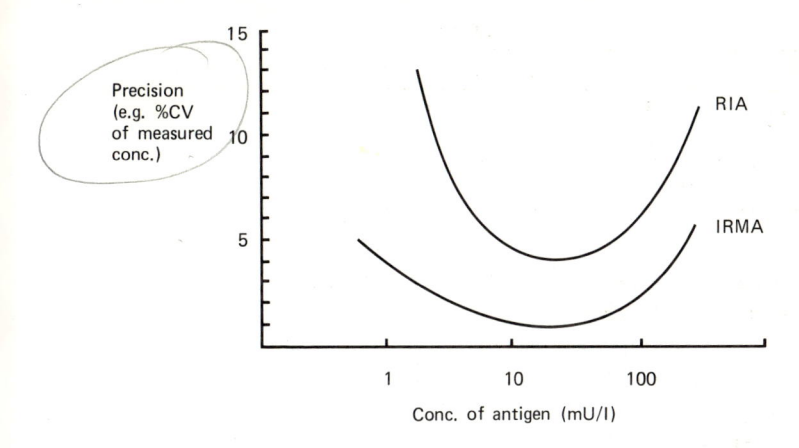

Figure 4.10 *Comparison of the precision profiles for a radioimmunoassay and for an immunoradiometric assay. In this example of assays for human thyroid stimulating hormone (TSH), the precision of the IRMA is obviously better than the precision of the RIA. These profiles indicate the greater sensitivity and range of IRMA compared to RIA.*

more samples without the need for either serial dilution or repeat assays.

Effect of Non-specific Binding of Label

One important aspect of the immunoradiometric assay, often overlooked, is the effect of the non-specific binding of the radiolabel on the performance of the assay. The contribution of this 'blank' value to the overall measurement is proportionately greater at the low concentration end of the range, as illustrated in Figure 4.11. This means that errors, by contributing to the magnitude of the blank measurement, can have a considerable effect on the sensitivity of the assay. The significance of this in practical terms is seen in the washing step. Washing of the solid-phase bound radiolabelled antibody to remove any non-specific binding can be extremely beneficial in terms of enhancing the sensitivity. This beneficial effect is more marked in the immunometric system than in the immunoassay system. As a reflection of this effect, errors in counting, usually not very significant in most radioimmunoassays, can play a significant role in

52 *Immunoassay*

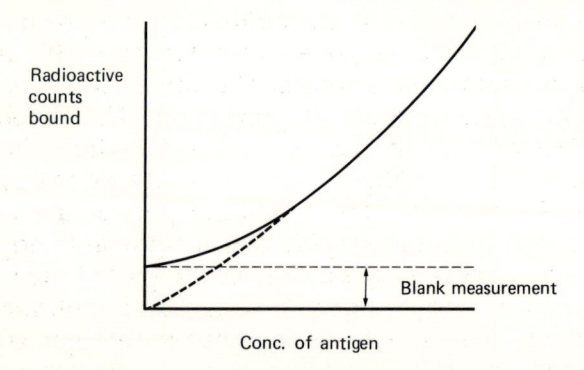

[Figure: curve showing radioactive counts bound vs conc. of antigen, with dashed line indicating blank measurement]

Figure 4.11 *Effect of non-specific binding in the relationship between bound radiolabelled antibody and concentration of antigen. A relatively high 'blank', affects the sensitivity; as the 'blank' increases, so sensitivity decreases.*

determining the potential sensitivity of an immunoradiometric assay. For this reason, it may prove necessary to count samples for a much longer time to achieve the maximum sensitivity of the assay.

The Biphasic Response

The immunoradiometric assay can give rise to a biphasic response. This biphasic response is often referred to as the 'hook' effect or the 'prozone' effect. The reaction between

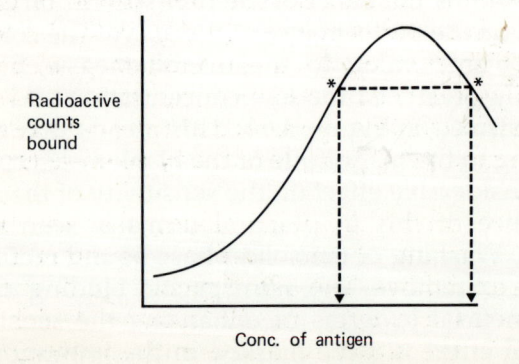

[Figure: biphasic curve showing radioactive counts bound vs conc. of antigen, with horizontal dashed line intersecting curve at two points marked with asterisks]

Figure 4.12 *The biphasic response in an immunometric assay. A particular level of bound radiolabelled antibody correlates with two different concentrations of antigen.*

antigen and antibody, as exemplified by the precipitin test, exhibits a biphasic response (see Chapter 10) and this general phenomenon is reflected in the 'hook' effect of the immunoradiometric assay (Figure 4.12). The 'hook' effect takes place at high antigen concentration where, in fact, in reaction terms, the antigen is in excess. As for the precipitin test (see Chapter 10), the ascending part of the response curve results from the specific reagent (the antibody) reacting in excess to the antigen. The second part of the response curve, the descending portion, begins and continues when the antibody is not in excess, i.e. when the antigen is present in sufficient quantity to react in excess to the antibody.

The problem that the biphasic response introduces into the assay is one of interpretation of results from high concentrations of antigen. As can be seen in Figure 4.12, these will be results in terms of counts from the solid-phase bound radiolabelled antibody which can be interpolated to two different concentrations of antigen. At very high concentrations of antigen the descending curve can reach a point equivalent to the values for very low concentrations. This is an extremely important point when the assay is applied to the investigation of antigens which may exist at very high levels; for example, in some pathological situations where tumours can secrete amounts many times that found normally.

Where it is a problem, the biphasic response can be reduced or eliminated. The sequential addition of reagents mentioned earlier in this chapter (p. 44), with the removal of unreacted species between each reagent addition by washing, will usually eliminate the 'hook' and replace it with a plateau. Although this does increase the technical complexity of the method, it will remove any possible ambiguity in the result.

It should, of course, be remembered that the biphasic response is a result of multivalency reactions between antigens and antibodies. The use of monospecific antibodies directed towards a single, unique epitope, which is not repeated within the structure of the antigen, would theoretically eliminate any multivalent reactions, providing the solid-phase antibody has a specificity for a different epitope to the epitope binding of the radiolabelled antibody.

Further Reading

Hales C. N., Woodhead J. S. (1980). Labelled antibodies and their use in the immunoradiometric assay. In: *Methods in Enzymology, Vol. 70: Immunochemical Techniques, Part A*. London: Academic Press.

Merrett T. G., Merrett J. (1980). The RAST principle and the use of mixed-allergen RAST as a screening test of IgG-mediated allergies. In: *Methods in Enzymology, Vol. 70: Immunochemical Techniques, Part A*. London: Academic Press.

Parratt D., McKenzie H., Nielson K. H., Cobb S. J. (1982). *Radioimmunoassay of Antibody and its Clinical Applications*. New York: John Wiley & Sons.

CHAPTER FIVE

Antibodies: Polyclonal and Monoclonal

Introduction

The antibody as the specific reagent in immunoassay is crucial to performance. An antiserum with high specificity and a high affinity constant (K value) will confer the attributes of good specificity and sensitivity on any assay in which it is used. As the quality of the antibody will be more relevant to assay performance than the quality of any other reagent, it will be useful to critically evaluate the techniques used to produce and prepare antibodies.

The Immune Response

The production of antibodies is a specific event in the more general phenomenon known as the immune response. The immune response is basically a series of related events (Figure 5.1) in a living animal in response to the presence of a substance considered to be alien or foreign to that particular system. Sophisticated immune responses are found widely throughout the vertebrate world, particularly in mammals.

Following immunisation or stimulation of the immune response with an immunogen (an immunogen is that which will stimulate the immune system), antibodies produced by the B lymphocytes will circulate in the blood system and may well be present for periods of time from weeks to months. Serum taken from the blood of an immunised animal is called antiserum. The antiserum will contain the antibodies which would comprise only a small proportion, up to 1%, of the total serum proteins.

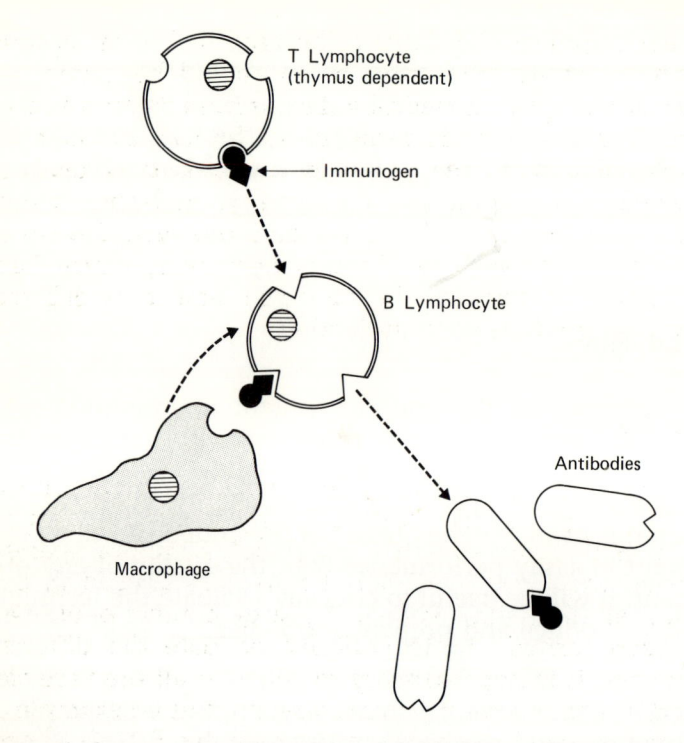

Figure 5.1 Cellular and molecular basis of the immune response; through the reaction of antigens with specific binding receptors on the cell surface, specific B lymphocytes are stimulated to both secrete specific immunoglobulins (antibodies), and to multiply in large numbers. Appropriate and efficient stimulation of the B lymphocytes is assisted by T lymphocytes reacting with immunogen, also through surface receptors. Reaction of immunogen with macrophages also stimulates specific B lymphocytes.

Immunogen

A distinction can be made between the immunogen, that which stimulates the immune response, and the antigen, that which reacts immunologically with the antibody. In some circumstances the same molecule may act as both immunogen and antigen, but this is certainly not always the case. A protein or peptide with a molecular weight of approximately 5000 or greater will generally act as an immunogen. For other substances such as polysaccharides, the minimum molecular weight required to induce an immune response may have to be greater. For an optimal immune response, the immunogen should be introduced into an animal phylogenetically distant from its own species origin. If a response is required to human proteins for example, rabbits or sheep could be immunised. It has been suggested that evolutionary conservative molecules would not be expected to make good immunogens. However, many substances such as pituitary hormones, which have considerable portions of the molecule similar in different species, do produce good antibodies.

Immunisation

There are many reported schedules for successful immunisation. The largest single variable in any immunisation programme is the animal, either individual, family or species. However, these must generally be taken as anecdotal, and very few studies with a sufficiently large number of animals have been carried out to critically evaluate the different procedures. It is not necessary to consider all the variables connected with successful immunisation, but an example of a commonly used method is given in Table 5.1. The most frequently used animals for producing antisera have been rabbits, sheep, guinea pigs, goats, swine, horses and donkeys. Seventy per cent of human blood donors have been

Table 5.1
Immunisation Schedule

---
100 µg Antigen in 0·5 ml physiological saline
Add 1ml Freunds complete adjuvant
Homogenise
Inject three or four sites subcutaneously on back of animal
    Leave for 2–3 weeks
Bleed for testing
    Leave for 3–4 weeks
Repeat injections (except replace complete adjuvant with incomplete)
    Leave for 2–3 weeks
Bleed for testing
    Leave for 3–4 weeks
Repeat injections or immunologically rest

Continue until satisfactory antiserum obtained
---

found to have antibodies in their serum which react with immunoglobulin from cow, sheep, goat and guinea pig and only to a much smaller extent with those from horse, swine and rabbits. So when producing antisera for assay of human material, it might be useful to select the latter species first.

With persistence and patience, it is usually possible to produce antibodies to even the most weakly immunogenic substances. Where the initial responses are low, it can be useful to 'immunologically rest' the animal for a period of a few months before continuing with the immunisation schedule. This simply means that the animal is not immunised for the period of 'immunological rest' and then the injections are started again.

Hapten Principle

Where it is necessary to produce an antiserum to a substance which is not immunogenic itself, it becomes necessary to conjugate the substance to something that is immunogenic, even if only weakly so. The low molecular weight substances which react with an antibody raised against the immunogenic conjugate are called haptens. Invoking this principle has led to the production of a vast number of antisera to small molecules like steroids, peptides, drugs and nucleotides. To covalently couple a hapten to a 'carrier' immunogen, the hapten must possess a reactive chemical group such as an amino group ($-NH_2$) or a carboxylic group ($-COOH$). Where no reactive group exists, it is necessary to use an analogue or derivative with a reactive group. Providing there is a degree of homogeneity between the analogue and the hapten, the resulting antibody will react appropriately with the hapten.

Testing of Antisera

Samples of antisera are most frequently tested by measuring the titre. The titre is given by measuring the amount of labelled antigen bound by varying the dilution of the antiserum (Figure 5.2). Although the titre of an antiserum

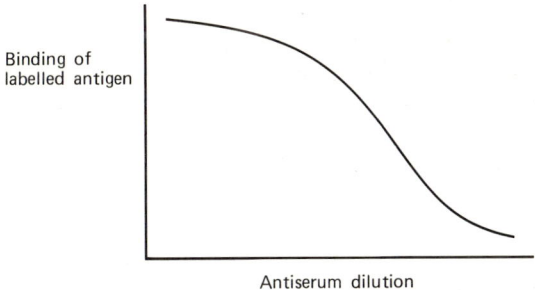

Figure 5.2 *The titre of an antiserum; the binding of a small amount of labelled antigen at different dilutions of an antiserum indicates the potential level of antibodies. For a given binding of labelled antigen, a low titre is indicated by a higher concentration of antiserum (low dilution), and a high titre by a lower concentration of antiserum (high dilution).*

will indicate the presence of antibodies, it will say little about quality. A defined titre could result from a high concentration of low affinity antibodies or equally from a low concentration of high affinity antibodies. A similar titre will also arise from an infinite number of combinations between these two extremes. As already stated, the quality, and in particular the affinity, of the antiserum is critical in terms of the potential performance of the assay. It thus becomes important to select an antiserum from various test bleeds using more appropriate information. Whilst it may not be practical to fully assess all test bleeds, it is often possible to get the necessary information using a minimum of additional work.

Information on the sensitivity may be gained by carrying out titration of the antiserum in the presence of a minimum concentration of antigen and then comparing it with the original titre as in Figure 5.3. A reduction of titre could indicate satisfactory sensitivity.

Some information on specificity can also be obtained from titration curves. For this, the titration of antiserum is carried out in the presence of a large concentration of a known cross reactant, or the cross reactant considered to give rise to most of the problems. This test is illustrated in Figure 5.4, where similar titres would indicate high specificity.

The equilibrium constant, or K value, often the most useful parameter, can sometimes be assessed by the shape of

60 *Immunoassay*

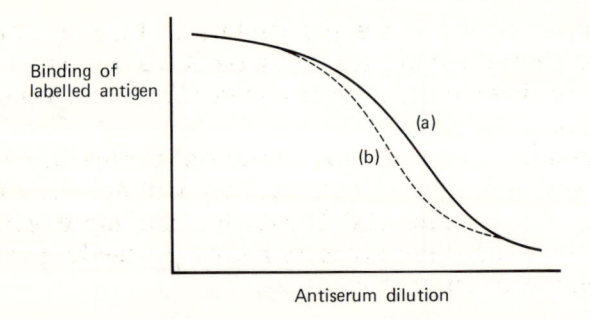

Figure 5.3 *Sensitivity as measured by the titration curve; displacement of the titration curve in the presence of a fixed amount of unlabelled antigen (b), from the titre in the absence of unlabelled antigen (a), indicates the required sensitivity.*

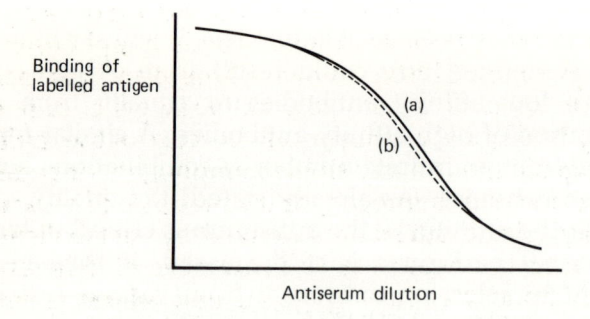

Figure 5.4 *Specificity as measured by the titration curve; similar titres obtained in the presence of a fixed amount of a known cross-reacting molecule (b), and in its absence (a), indicates specificity of the antiserum.*

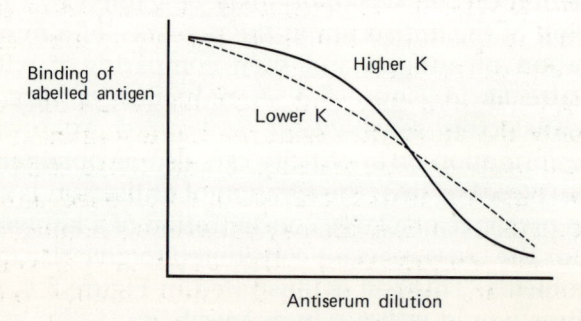

Figure 5.5 *Affinity (K) as measured by the titration curve; relative affinities are sometimes indicated by the slope of the titration curve.*

the titration curve. A steeper decline in titre, as the antiserum is diluted, indicates a higher K value, and a more shallow decline would indicate a lower K value, as shown in Figure 5.5.

The results obtained from titration curves are strictly relative and subjective. However, they will help in selecting the most appropriate test bleeds for the more extensive testing that is usually necessary before proceeding with the development of an immunoassay.

Heterogeneity of Antibodies in Antisera

Every specific antibody produced by the immune system in response to any given immunogen will come from a lymphocyte line derived from an original single lymphocyte. Each lymphocyte line will have its own intrinsic and independent capacity to produce a particular antibody genetically determined by its original precursor cell. Because of the multiplicity of antigenic sites on any single immunogen, or because of impurities in the immunogen, or the presence of a number of chemically related substances derived by metabolism once injected into the animal, a large number of different and distinct lymphocytes may be stimulated following immunisation. As a consequence, antisera invariably contain a heterogenous mixture of different antibodies of varying specificity and affinity. They also usually contain a mixture of immunoglobulin classes. There is evidence to suggest that the genetic expression for antibodies undergoes a higher than normal frequency of mutation, leading to even greater heterogeneity of molecular species.

At a high dilution, that is at a low concentration, of the antisera only the antibodies with the highest affinities will, for practical purposes, be reacting. Under these conditions, and in combination with highly purified labelled antigens, the heterogeneous antiserum may behave as a homogeneous reagent in an immunoassay. The potential problems of heterogeneity are often reduced where highly purified immunogens are available for immunisation and purified antigens are available for labelling. The heterogeneity indicates the potential advantage gained by appropriate purification of the labelled antigen before use in the immunoassay. In these circumstances, the purified labelled antigen would monitor the reaction with only a small population of specific antibodies.

A recent refinement of some considerable interest has been the production of antibodies derived from a single cell line, the monoclonal antibody. Since the advent of monoclonal antibodies, the antibodies in conventional antisera have been called polyclonal.

Monoclonal Antibodies

Lymphocytes are notoriously difficult to culture and so do not lend themselves to selection *in vitro*. However, following the pioneering work of Harris and his co-workers in the 1960s, and subsequent developments to the definitive work of Kohler and Milstein in 1975, it was found that the fusion of specific lymphocytes with myeloma cells yielded hybrid cells that were stable *in vitro* and could be cultured. These hybridoma cells continued to produce the specific antibody predefined by the original lymphocyte cell. The general technique for the production of monoclonal antibodies is given in Figure 5.6.

Stimulated B lymphocytes are induced in an animal by conventional immunisation schedules. The mouse is chosen for this, as it is necessary for the lymphocytes to be compatible with the myeloma strain, and most successful myelomas have been derived from mice. When the immunised mouse is optimally secreting antibodies, it is sacrificed and the spleen is homogenised to give a cell suspension containing the active lymphocytes. A fusion of lymphocytes and myeloma cells is induced by polyethylene glycol (the most successful of fusion agents used so far) and the fused cells are selected from the unfused lymphocytes and the unfused myeloma cells. Selection is carried out in a medium (HAT—Hypoxanthine-Aminopteridin-Thyronidine) which is essentially toxic to the myeloma, a mutant devoid of certain enzymes, but in which the hybridoma survives as it contains the enzymes genetically derived from lymphocytes. The unfused lymphocytes do not survive in culture. This

Antibodies: Polyclonal and Monoclonal 63

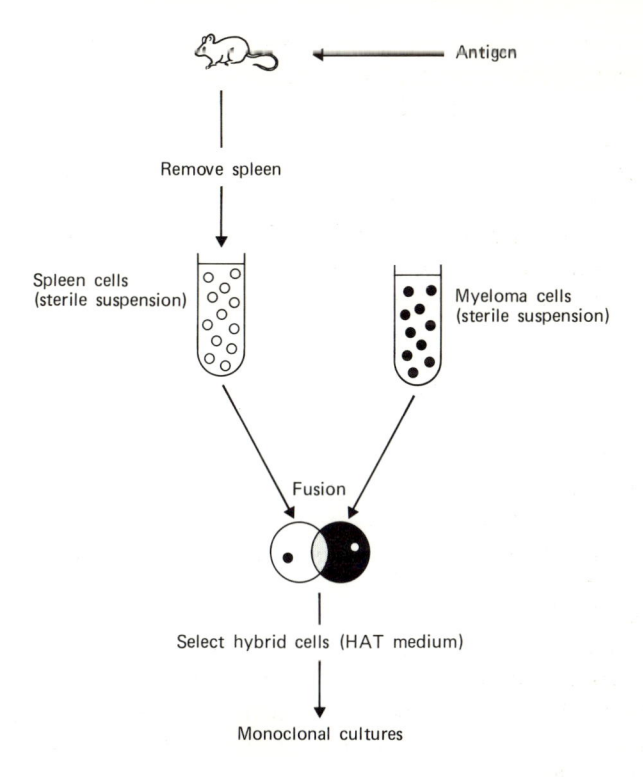

Figure 5.6 *Production of monoclonal antibodies.*

ability to select hybridomas by culture is obviously a key process in the practical success of the technique. Surviving hybridomas are plated out in agar and cultured to give single cell clones. These clones are cultured, and the culture medium is tested for the presence of antibodies. Positive clones are recloned and cultured for further investigation. A portion of any positive clone can also be frozen, in liquid nitrogen, to avoid any possible loss of the cell line in culture. As the selected hybridoma cultures are each derived from a single cell, the antibody secreted should be of a predefined nature. Due to stability of the frozen cell lines and stability of growth in appropriate culture medium, the supply of antibody is considered to be permanent. This means that any given monoclonal antibody is constantly available with a consistent and a predefined specificity. This means that antibodies can have the essential qualities that are common for many other analytical reagents.

Problems of Monoclonal Antibody Production

Although monoclonal antibodies offer considerable and obvious advantages, and, indeed, represent a considerable advance in the application of immunoassay methods, one should not underestimate the level of expertise required to produce them or, indeed, the amount of work necessary to screen all the clones, of which only a few will secrete the appropriate antibodies.

Perhaps, for the very reason that monoclonal antibodies appear to be the answer to many problems, special emphasis should be made in detailing the practical problems involved in the production of monoclonal antibodies.

The first major difficulty is with contamination. Contamination with bacteria, fungi or mycoplasma have all caused considerable difficulties, and work in some groups has been held up for many months until the infection has been eliminated. If the cell line gets infected, this may well mean a complete loss. For this reason alone, production of monoclonal antibodies should be left to those groups with the necessary expertise.

Another important aspect of monoclonal antibody production is the success rate of the fusion step. The ratio of the number of lymphocytes to the number of successfully fused hybridomas may fall by a factor of 10^4 to 10^5. The implication here is that those lymphocytes secreting antibodies relevant to the required immunogen will also fall by a similar factor. This could give one antibody producing hybridoma for every 10 000 to 100 000 relevant lymphocytes. Given that there is some evidence to suggest that actively-secreting lymphocytes can be favourably selected (by a factor of 10) in the fusion step, there would still be a considerable loss of potential antibodies. In theory, this could mean that 10 000 to 100 000 times as many experiments would be necessary to be sure of producing all the antibodies produced *in vivo*. Certainly, one would not expect to find antibodies from just one screening of a fusion experiment that are as good as those available from conventional antisera. A considerable amount of work is definitely involved in the production of most useful monoclonal antibodies.

For some antigens, the species choice for monoclonal antibody production (the mouse) may not be appropriate. Some antigens are relatively weak immunogens in the mouse, and this could limit the full potential of monoclonal antibodies, until myeloma strains derived from other species are available.

Many monoclonal antibodies lack the normal precipitating behaviour found for polyclonal antisera. This is almost certainly a reflection of the monospecificity of the monoclonal antibody. The conventional precipitate, being a three-dimensional lattice of antibodies and antigens, requires heterogeneity of binding sites and antibodies to provide maximum cross-linking. Presumably, one solution to this difficulty would be to mix different monoclonal antibodies to give the necessary heterogeneity.

Some monoclonal antibodies are very labile, and activity may be lost on freezing and thawing, or simply on long-term storage.

One additional aspect to be considered, is the frequent need to purify a monoclonal antibody from monoclonal culture medium or the murine ascites fluid. This would be necessary if use is to be made of the monoclonal antibody as a purified reagent for labelling, e.g. in an immunometric assay.

Advantages of Monoclonal Antibody Production

In addition to the advantages already mentioned, i.e. the perpetual production of a predefined and homogeneous reagent, the production of monoclonal antibody offers one considerable advantage. It is extremely useful for the production of specific antibodies to impure or mixed immunogens (see Figure 5.7). For example, raising specific antibodies to cells, one cell type can have many antigenic sites on its surface membranes, many of which might be common to other cell types. Isolation of membrane antigens may be difficult and, of course, loss of complete membrane structures may lead to a change in the tertiary structure of the antigen. The hybridoma technique has been very useful in solving these problems, and has yielded many cell-type specific antibodies. Monoclonal antibodies, raised against impure antigens, have been used subsequently in the large-scale purification of the antigen; for example, interferon, or indeed the cell, as in the removal of leukaemic cells from bone marrow.

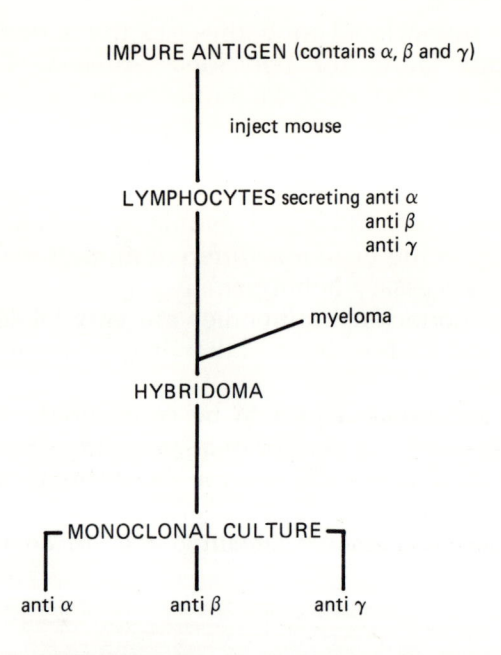

```
        IMPURE ANTIGEN (contains α, β and γ)
                     |
                inject mouse
                     |
        LYMPHOCYTES secreting anti α
                              anti β
                              anti γ
                     |
                     |_____ myeloma
                     |
                 HYBRIDOMA
                     |
              ┌─ MONOCLONAL CULTURE ─┐
              |          |           |
           anti α      anti β      anti γ
```

Figure 5.7 *Principle of producing specific antibodies from a heterogenous mixture of antigens through monoclonal culture.*

Because of the various limitations and problems with monoclonal antibody production, there are many situations where other approaches may be necessary or desirable. Purification of antibodies by affinity chromatography and immunisation with precipitates from crossed immunoelectrophoresis are two techniques that have offered considerable advantages over the years, and the potential of these approaches should not be underestimated.

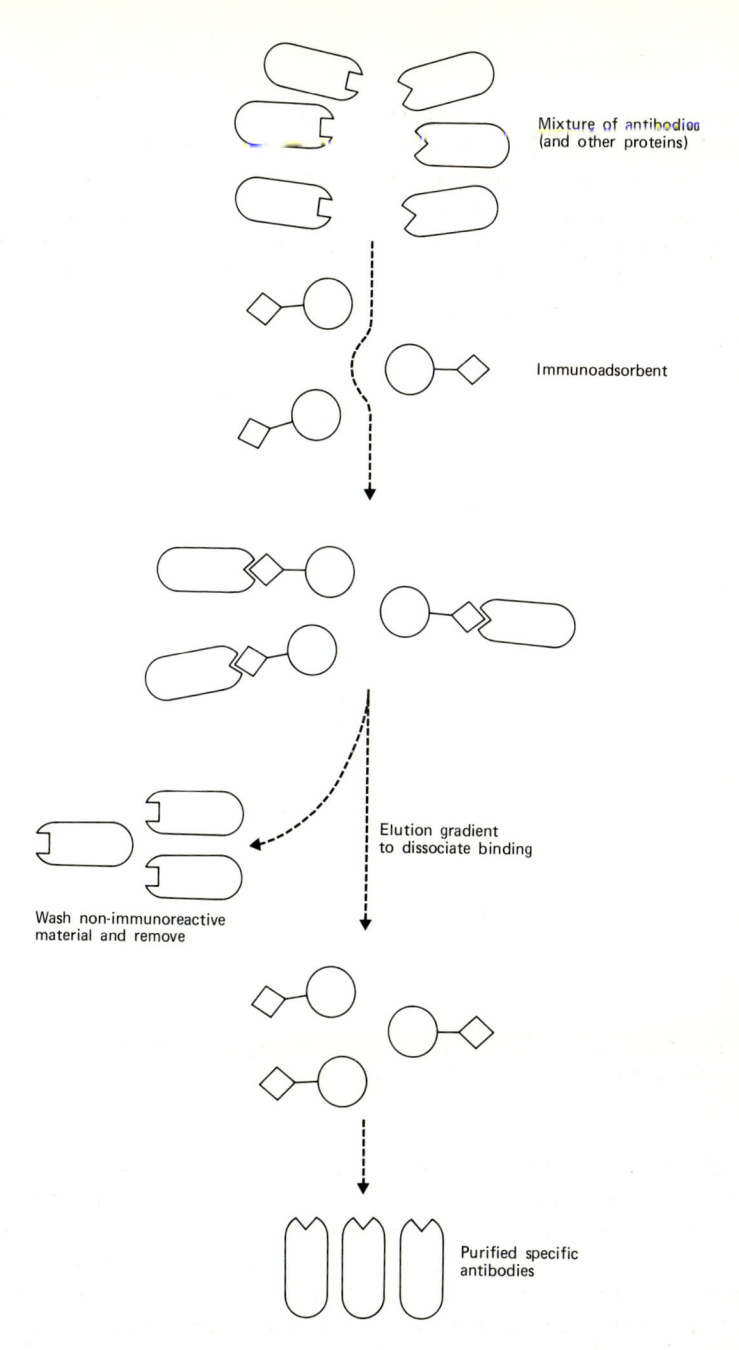

Figure 5.8 *Affinity chromatography of immunoglobulins to produce specific antibodies.*

Purification of Antibodies by Affinity Chromatography

In the original immunoradiometric assay of Miles and Hales in 1968, the labelled antibodies were purified by adsorption to a solid-phase antigen (the immunosorbent), and subsequent elution by reducing the pH. This method produced antibodies with defined specificity but, because of the low yields, it was very costly in terms of antisera. In 1974, Woodhead considerably improved the method by eluting antibodies with a combination of pH reduction and a polar reducing reagent, dimethylformamide. Yields were increased 10- to 50-fold. The general method of affinity chromatography to purify antibodies, whilst not expected to isolate 'monoclonal' antibodies, should be capable of isolating 'isotypic' antibodies, i.e. a population of antibodies reacting with a single antigenic site. Figure 5.8 shows, in

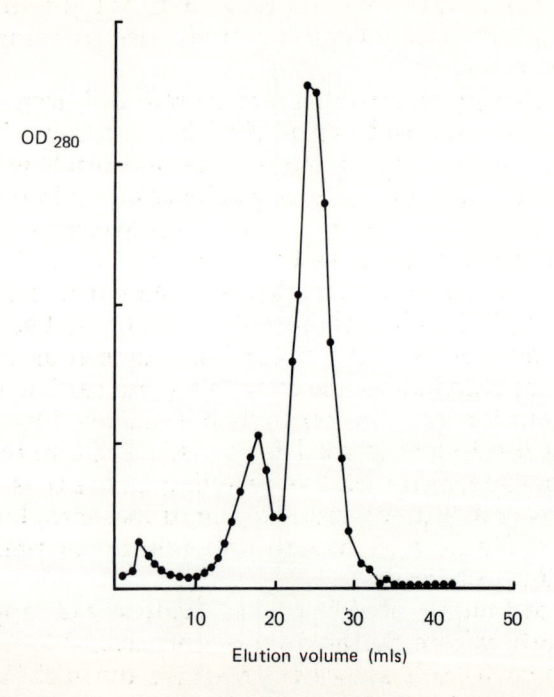

Figure 5.9 *Purification of antibodies following affinity chromatography; elution profile of antibodies (anti-human TSH) from immunosorbent (Sepharose 4B linked to human TSH) using a pH gradient (pH 7.0 to pH 3.0) in 20% acetonitrile.*

diagrammatic form, the isolation of antibodies by affinity chromatography, and Figure 5.9 shows the elution profile from a specific purification using affinity chromatography. By judicious use of various parameters, e.g. pH reduction, polar reducing reagents and various cross reactants, it is possible to introduce very subtle changes during the elution from the immunosorbent, separating the antibodies into more and more homogeneous groups. This method could have an increasing use for the preparation of immunological reagents with improved specificity and affinity, often with a predefined functional activity.

Immunisation with Immunoprecipitates

Immunisation with specific antibody-antigen precipitates isolated from other antigen precipitates has been used since 1964 to produce monospecific antibodies to complex antigenic mixtures.

In the first place, an antiserum is produced from an animal immunised with crude unpurified immunogens. This antiserum is usually very heterogeneous and reacts with all the components present in the original mixture of immunogens. The crude mixture of immunogens is separated and precipitated by crossed immunoelectrophoresis in gels (see p. 118, Chapter 10). An example of this is shown in Figure 5.10. Each precipitation line represents a distinct antigen precipitated by antibodies in the original heterogeneous antiserum. A distinct precipitation line containing one particular antigen is cut from the gel. The precipitate is removed by washing, and this precipitate is used for subsequent immunisations. The monospecificity of the resulting antisera is demonstrated by subsequent crossed immunoelectrophoresis, as shown in Figure 5.11, where only one major precipitation line is now observed.

This technique obviously has widespread application, particularly where the antigen is only available in a crude form, such as cell sonicates. Because the technique only requires very small amounts of antigen, it would be especially useful where supplies of the antigen are limited, or particularly expensive.

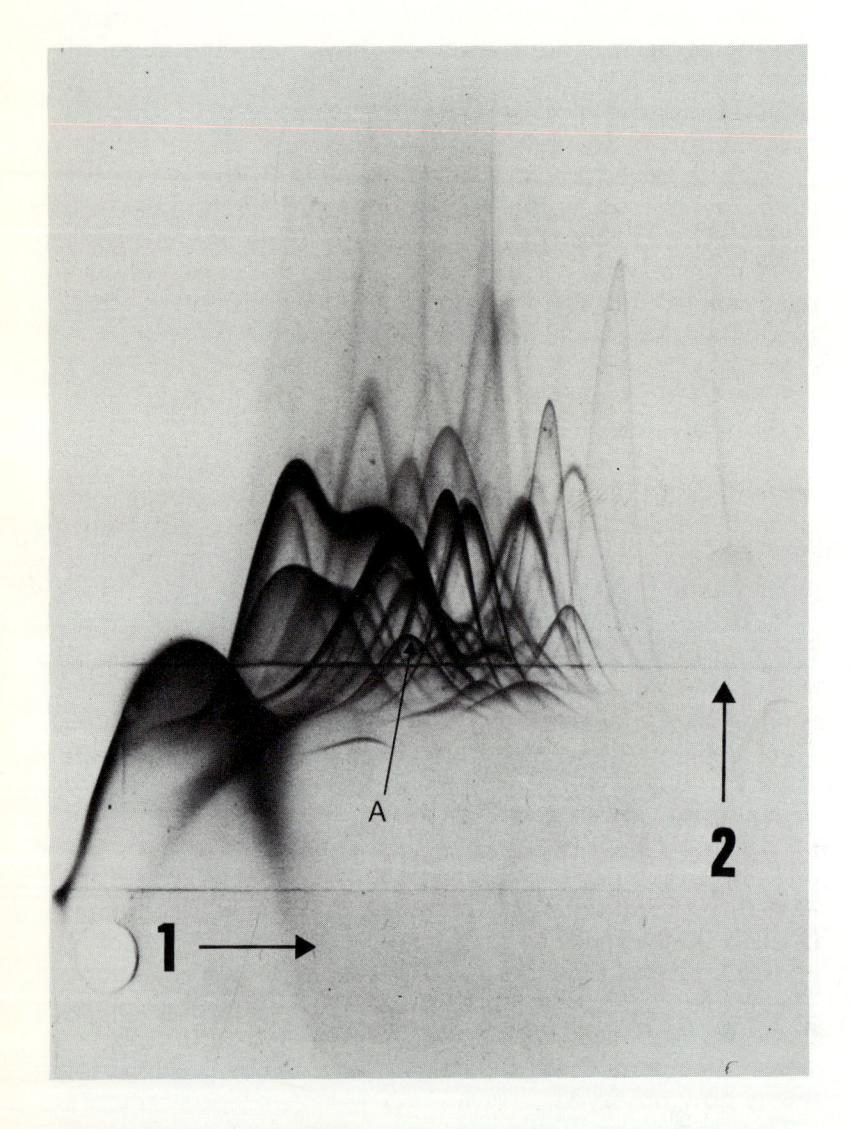

Figure 5.10 Crossed immunoelectrophoresis of a crude antigen mixture precipitated with its respective antiserum.

(a) Crude antigen mixture, prepared from culture of a tubercle bacillus (BCG), has been separated in one dimension (→1) and then electrophoresed into a gel (→2) containing a polyvalent anti-BCG. More than 50 different antigenic components are present and one specific antigen (A) is identified.

Antibodies: Polyclonal and Monoclonal 71

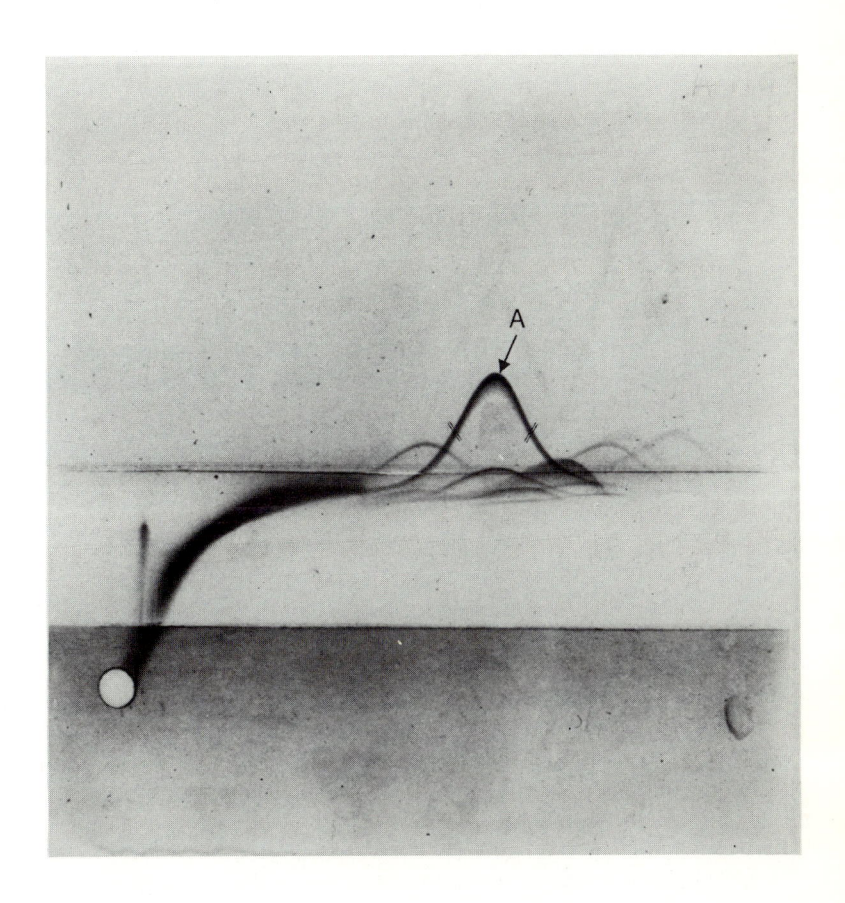

(b) Crossed immunoelectrophoresis of a less crude BCG fraction gives rise to an immunoprecipitate for antigen 'A', free from other precipitin lines. The specific precipitate is cut out of the gel as indicated and used for immunisation. A highly specific antiserum is obtained (see Figure 5.11).

(Photographs by courtesy of Professor M Harboe, Rikshospitalet, Oslo.)

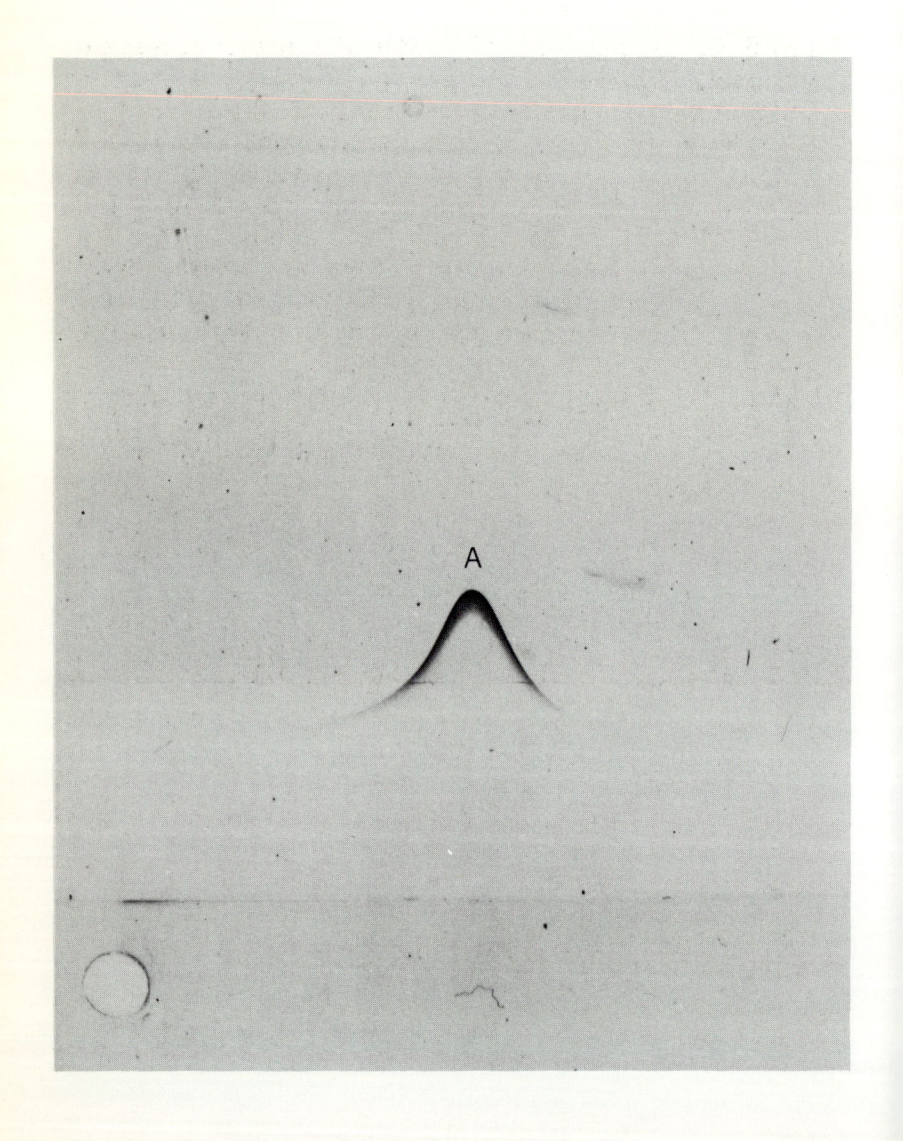

Figure 5.11 *Crossed immunoelectrophoresis of the same crude antigen mixture (Figure 5.10a) precipitated with antiserum raised against the isolated immunoprecipitate of antigen 'A' (see Figure 5.10b).*

Further Reading

Hurn B. A. L., Chantler S. M. (1980). Production of reagent antibodies. In: *Methods in enzymology, Vol. 70: Immunochemical Techniques, Part A.* London: Academic Press.

Harboe M., Closs O. (1983). Immunization with precipitates obtained by crossed immunoelectrophoresis. In: *Handbook of Immunoprecipitation-in-Gel Techniques.* (Axelsen N. H., ed.) Oxford: Blackwell Scientific Publications.

Marchalonis J. J. (1982). Structure of antibodies and usefulness to non-immunologists. In: *Antibody as a Tool: The Applications of Immunochemistry.* New York: John Wiley & Sons.

McMichael A. J., Fabre J. W., eds. (1982). *Monoclonal Antibodies in Clinical Medicine.* London: Academic Press.

Milstein C. (1980). Monoclonal antibodies. *Scientific American;* **243**(4): 56–105.

Various authors (1981). Production of antibodies. In: *Methods in Enzymology, Vol. 73: Immunochemical Techniques, Part B, Section I.* London: Academic Press.

Warr G. W. (1982). In: *Antibody as a Tool: The Applications of Immunochemistry.* New York: John Wiley & Sons.

CHAPTER SIX

Enzyme-Labelled Immunoassay Methods

Introduction

The publication in 1966 of methods for labelling immunological reagents with enzymes provided a stimulus for the rapid growth of immunoassay methods using the enzymic reaction as a detection system for the discrimination of antigen or antibody.

The basis of enzyme labels is illustrated in Figure 6.1. Analogous to the use of radioisotopes, enzymes may be linked as labels to either the antigen or the antibody. The enzyme-labelled assay may also be categorised into either immunoassay (limited reagent) or immunometric (excess reagent) techniques.

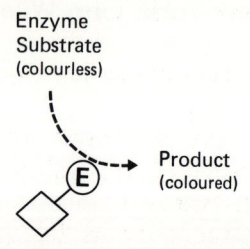

Figure 6.1 *The use of an enzyme to label immunological reagents. The amount of product (or colour) is proportional to the concentration of enzyme, which in turn is proportional to the concentration of either antigen or antibody, depending on which is labelled.*

The Enzyme Immunoassay (limited reagent)

The most sensitive and precise enzyme immunoassays are usually carried out with immobilised antibody, i.e. attached to either a particulate solid phase, adsorbed to a plastic bead, or adsorbed to the plastic wall of the reaction tube. With a limiting concentration of antibody and varying concen-

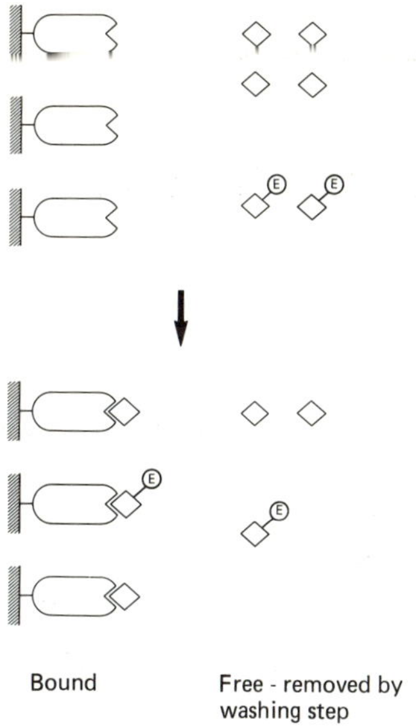

Figure 6.2 *Enzyme immunoassay; solid-phase antibody (limited concentration) reacts with the antigen and enzyme-labelled antigen.* The relationship between bound enzyme and concentration of antigen is the same as for bound counts and antigen concentration in RIA (Figure 2.3, p. 16).

trations of antigen, enzyme-labelled antigen will be bound in an inverse proportion (Figure 6.2). With an immobilised antibody, the free fraction of antigen and enzyme-labelled antigen are easily separated. It is also easy to wash the bound antigen fraction before measuring enzyme activity. This washing step is often very useful in removing factors that would otherwise interfere in the accurate measurement of enzyme activity. Interfering factors can be expected to be much more dominant if the sample is a complex biological fluid such as serum, in which many substances relevant to particular enzyme reactions, e.g. substrates or cofactors, exist.

Homogeneous Assays

A particular advantage of the enzyme-labelled immunoassay methods, not applicable to the use of radioisotopic labels, is that assays may be carried out without the use of separation techniques or precipitation to separate the free and bound fractions. These assays are usually referred to as homogeneous immunoassay methods. Immunoassay methods which rely on some form of separation of the fractions are referred to as heterogeneous in this terminology.

Homogeneous enzyme immunoassay methods arise because the binding of antibody and antigen interfere in some way with the enzymic reaction of the enzyme label. This interference is usually reflected by an inhibition of the enzymic reaction (Figure 6.3). The inhibition of the enzyme is most likely to occur through steric hindrance of substrate binding, by the presence of the large molecular size of the antibody, or perhaps through some change in three-dimensional configuration of the enzyme, leading to a reduction in its activity.

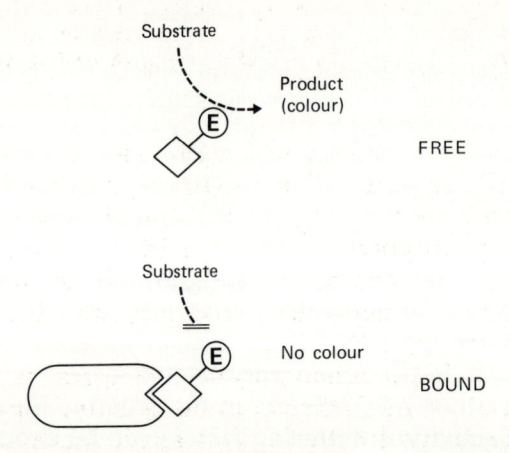

Figure 6.3 *An homogeneous enzyme immunoassay; in this assay a separation step is not necessary as the signal (enzyme reaction) is reduced or eliminated by antibody binding.*

The principle of homogeneous enzyme assays has been applied almost exclusively to the measurement of small molecular weight substances, where the enzyme is conjugated to the antigen. It was found originally that the principle was relatively ineffective where the antigen had a larger molecule size, as is the case when the antigen is a

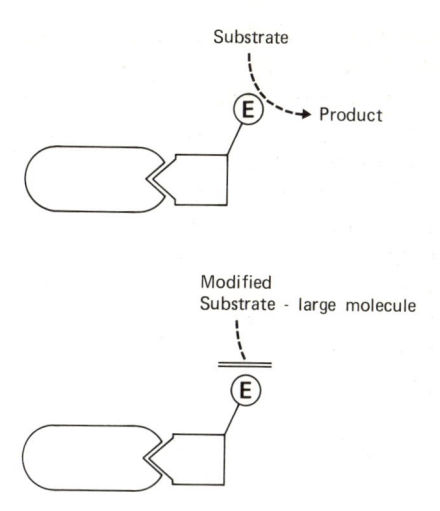

Figure 6.4 *Homogeneous enzyme immunoassay for large molecules; the conventional homogeneous enzyme immunoassay (Figure 6.3) is not usually effective for large molecules. However, if a suitably modified substrate, i.e. chromogenic substrate coupled to a large polymer, is used then antibody binding may inhibit the enzyme reaction.*

protein. However, subsequent work has shown that the principle will still be effective if a suitably modified substrate is used. Here, the chromogenic substrate is linked to a high molecular weight polymer. The inhibition of enzymic activity following the binding of the antibody to an enzyme-labelled protein antigen is almost certainly due to steric hindrances (Figure 6.4).

Binding of the antigen–enzyme conjugate by the antibody, instead of inhibiting enzyme activity, may actually increase the enzyme activity. This effect was noted when malate dehydrogenase was linked to the hapten thyroxine. A possible explanation for this phenomenon is that the antigen itself inhibited the enzyme in some way, and the inhibitory effect was removed when the antigen was bound to the antibody.

All these homogeneous assays are of the immunoassay type, i.e. limited reagent. With proportionately increasing concentration of antigen, there will be less binding of the enzyme–antigen conjugate, with the corresponding change either in inhibition of, or increase in, enzymic activity.

Enzyme Immunoassay with Labelled Antibody

Another example of an enzyme immunoassay, but with a labelled antibody rather than the conventional labelled antigen, is illustrated in Figure 6.5. Essentially, the method depends on the distribution of a limited amount of enzyme-labelled antibody between an immobilised antigen, prepared for the assay, and the antigen in the sample or standard. Maximum binding of the labelled antibody to the immobilised antigen will take place in the absence of antigen to be measured. As the concentration of antigen to be measured increases, so the amount of bound labelled antibody will proportionately decrease.

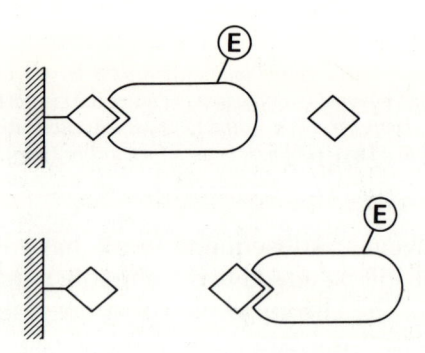

Figure 6.5 *Immunoassay with enzyme-labelled antibody; the labelled antibody binds to either the solid-phase antigen or the antigen in the sample. As the antigen concentration from the sample increases, so labelled antibody on the solid-phase decreases.*

Enzyme-Labelled Immunometric Assays

Antigens can be measured by immunometric assays using enzyme-labelled antibodies. These assays are invariably heterogeneous assays requiring a separation step. Because a washing step is a convenient way to remove interference in the final estimation of enzyme activity, these assays are conventionally carried out with a solid-phase component, particularly with one component attached to the test tube wall.

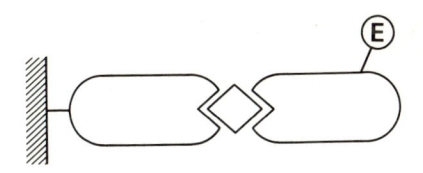

Figure 6.6 *Immunometric assay with enzyme-labelled antibody; antigen, bound by the solid-phase antibody, is measured by the binding of labelled antibody, i.e. analogous to the 'two site' immunoradiometric assay (Figure 4.3, p. 43), and conventionally known as ELISA.*

The basic assay is performed by reacting the antigen with an immobilised antibody present in the reaction in excess. The concentration of antigen is then determined by the addition of an enzyme-labelled antibody, once again in excess (Figure 6.6).

This basic immunometric assay is usually referred to in the literature as ELISA—the enzyme linked immunosorbent assay. ELISA has been used very successfully to measure and monitor the presence of antibodies in biological fluids, especially blood. In this variant of ELISA, the immunosorbent is an immobilised antigen relevant to the particular antibody to be measured. After reacting the immobilised antigen with the varying concentrations of antibodies present in samples, the bound antibodies are detected following a subsequent reaction with an enzyme-labelled anti-immunoglobulin antibody (Figure 6.7).

Enzyme-labelled
anti-immunoglobulin
(second antibody)

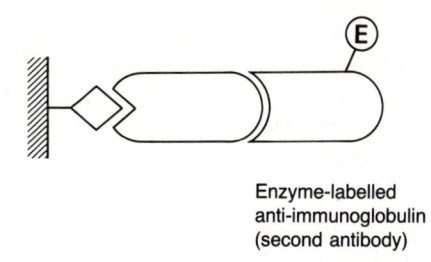

Figure 6.7 *ELISA for measuring antibodies; antibodies bound by a solid-phase antigen are measured by a labelled anti-immunoglobulin. This assay is frequently used to monitor infectious diseases by measuring circulating specific antibodies.*

Indirect Labelling

As with immunoradiometric assays, there are also variations of the ELISA technique which use indirect labelling. The specific antibody responsible for quantitation is not labelled directly by conjugation to an enzyme but is labelled indirectly by a second reaction with an anti-immunoglobulin antibody, itself conjugated to an enzyme. As before (see p. 42, Chapter 4), if this technique is used in an assay dependent on an immobilised antibody (as in Figure 6.6), the immobilised antibody should come from a different species to that from which was taken the antibody to carry the indirect label.

The Enzyme

The enzyme of choice should be selected primarily on the basis of three parameters.

1) The enzyme should have a high turnover rate of substrate to product, thus maximising the amplification of measurement or detection from the substance for assay to the final signal.

2) The product should be detected with maximum sensitivity. This clearly implies that the product signal should be absent in the substrate. In simple terms, this would mean that a colourless substrate gives rise to a coloured product.

3) The enzyme activity should be minimally susceptible to interference from factors likely to be present in the sample. These factors include pH, presence of common preservatives (some of which may inhabit the enzyme), enzyme cofactors, enzyme substrates or inhibitors and indeed other enzymes which may compete for the substrate. Obviously, sample interference will be less significant where immobilised reagents are used with washing steps. Enzymes used with varying success in enzyme-labelled immunoassay methods are listed in Table 6.1.

The enzymes malate dehydrogenase and glucose-6-phosphate dehydrogenase have been used extensively in the

Table 6.1
Enzymes used in Immunoassays

Enzyme	Source
Lysozyme	Hen egg white
Malate dehydrogenase	Pig heart mitochondria
Glucose-6-phosphate dehydrogenase	Bacterial (*Leuconostoc mesenteroides*)
Peroxidase	Horseradish
Glucose oxidase	*Aspergillus niger*
Alkaline phosphatase	*Escherichia coli* or veal intestine
β-Galactosidase	*Escherichia coli*

homogeneous enzyme immunoassays exemplified by the Syva EMIT (Enzyme Multiplied Immunoassay Technique) system. Both enzymes are monitored by the conversion of the cofactor NAD to $NADH_2$ in a spectrophotometer at 340 nm.

The enzymes most favoured in the ELISA method (Table 6.2) have been alkaline phosphatase and horseradish peroxidase. However, the use of β-galactosidase has several advantages, and its use is increasing. Activity of these three enzymes is measured by a colour development in a synthetic chromogenic substrate.

If a precise and accurate measurement is required, the colour is measured at an appropriate wavelength in a spectrophotometer. Frequently, the development of the colour is read by eye. Although this would imply a qualititative assay, it becomes quantitative by assaying each sample at a number of serial dilutions. The highest dilution to give a positive result is taken as a measure of potency.

Table 6.2
Enzyme Labels Commonly Used in ELISA

Enzyme	Substrate	Colour of product
Alkaline phosphatase	*p*-nitrophenylphosphate	Yellow
Horseradish peroxidase	*o*-phenylenediamine	Brown
β-Galactosidase*	*o*-nitrophenylphosphate (non-toxic)	Yellow

*Not inhibited by bacteriostatic agents.

82 Immunoassay

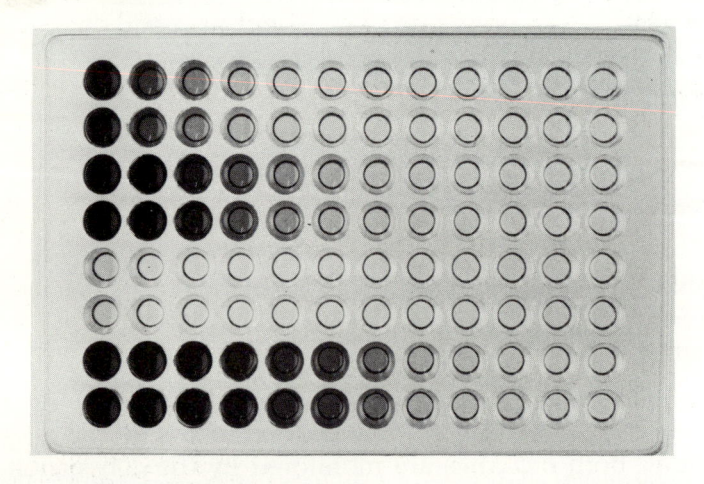

Figure 6.8 *ELISA in microtitre plate; plates consist of 96 wells and are made of polystyrene. Wells are coated with a specific antigen, e.g. malarial parasite, and samples can be assayed, in duplicate or in a series of dilutions, for presence of specific antibodies to the antigen. The presence of antibodies is measured by binding of an enzyme-labelled anti-immunoglobulin and subsequent colour development. (By courtesy of Dennis Bidwell.)*

Microtitre Plate

ELISA has exploited fully the use of the disposable microtitre plate with 96 wells (Figure 6.8). Either antigen or antibody can be adsorbed to the wall of each well by a simple coating procedure (Table 6.3). Subsequent washing steps and reagent addition steps become very easy using the microtitre system, particularly with the assistance of multihead pipet-

Table 6.3
Coating of Polystyrene Well

1. Pre-equilibrate wells at 4°C
2. Add 200 µl of carbonate buffer (pH 9·6, 0·05M) containing 1–10 µg protein/ml
3. Leave overnight at 4°C
4. Remove buffer and wash extensively

tes (Figure 6.9) or any of the automated and semi-automated pieces of equipment specially designed to handle the microtitre plate. Because of ease and simplicity, and the subsequent high throughput of microtitre plate, ELISA has become the method of choice for screening monoclonal antibody production cultures (see Chapter 5).

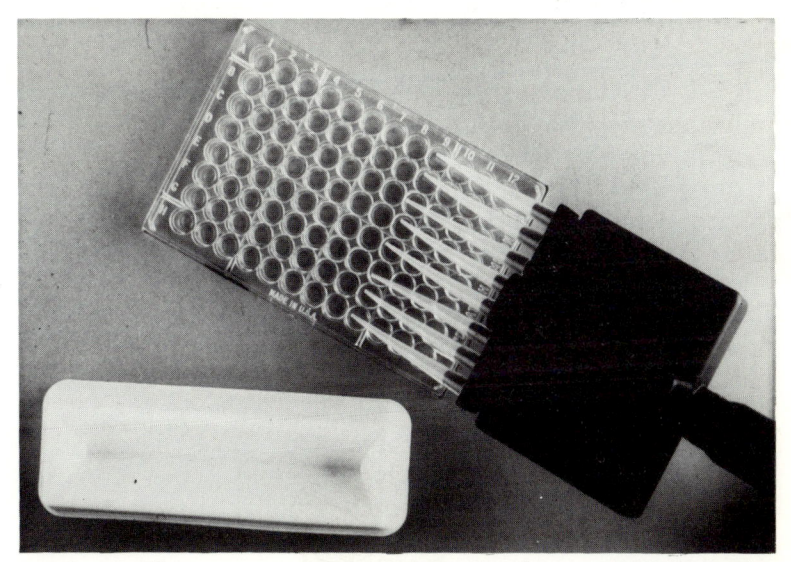

Figure 6.9 *Efficient reagent addition for microtitre plates; many devices, such as the multi-head pipette, can be used to improve the efficiency of ELISA. (By courtesy of Dennis Bidwell.)*

Preparation of Enzyme Label

The method used to covalently link the enzyme to the reagent can have an effect on the performance of the label and its suitability for the assay. A number of different methods have been used, but a few selected methods have been found to be particularly appropriate (Table 6.4).

Both the glutaraldehyde and periodate methods are relatively non-specific coupling procedures relying on activation of various reactive groups on both the enzyme and the reagent (antigen or antibody). These methods generally give

Table 6.4
Conjugation of Enzyme to Reagent

1. Glutaraldehyde—simultaneous (one step, i.e. add glutaraldehyde with both enzyme and reagent)
   —sequential (two step, i.e. activate enzyme with glutaraldehyde, then add reagent)
2. Periodate oxidation
3. Homobifunctional—N,N-o-phenylenedimaleimide
4. Heterobifunctional—m-maleimidobenzoyl-N-hydroxysuccinimide

rise to polymolecular polymers, comprising several molecules of both types. Loss of efficiency of enzyme activity after conjugation with these methods is common and may be as great as 90%. The product, being polymolecular, lacks precise definition and hence increases the possibility of batch-to-batch variation.

The periodate method couples through the carbohydrate portion of each molecule. As the carbohydrate part of the molecule is not usually involved in the active site of either the enzyme or the antibody, this method can give conjugates with less loss of activity.

More specific methods of conjugation have been used to good effect. The two examples given in Table 6.4, of a homobifunctional and a heterobifunctional reagent, tend to produce simple conjugates involving only a single molecule of both enzyme and reagent. Thus, the product has greater definition and usually retains full enzyme activity.

Following conjugation of enzyme to the reagent by any of these methods, the product will contain unreacted enzyme and reagent, in addition to the conjugate. These are removed before use in an assay as the presence of either will reduce the efficiency of the label. Purification by chromatography of the product (Figure 6.10) will also help remove any other impurities.

Salient Features of Enzyme-Labelled Immunoassay Methods

The most significant advantage of using enzyme labels is the potential long life of the labelled reagent. Providing the

OD$_{280}$

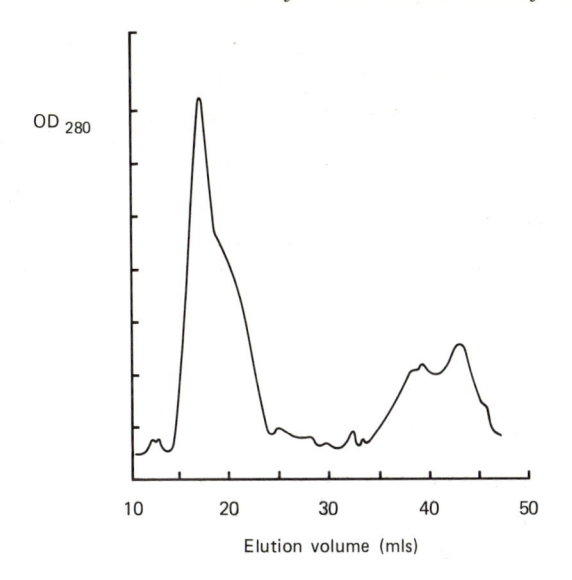

Elution volume (mls)

Figure 6.10 *Purification of an enzyme-labelled protein; the products of coupling albumin to horseradish peroxidase, using the sodium periodate method, are chromatographed on Sephadex G100 (45 × 1 cm) with phosphate buffer (pH 7.5, 0.05 mM) containing 0.9% sodium chloride and 0.1% sodium azide. The asymmetrical peak eluting between fractions 15 and 23 indicates the heterogeneous mixture of enzyme-albumin conjugates. Unconjugated enzyme and albumin elute later in the profile.*

enzyme conjugate and the enzyme substrate are stable, the basic reagents can last for several years.

As with radioimmunoassays, labelling the antigen with an enzyme usually requires the availability of highly purified antigen. However, unlike immunoradiometric assays, semipurified antibodies, or even unpurified antibodies, have been used successfully in applications of the ELISA technique. Crude immunoglobulin fractions of antisera are often used for labelling with enzymes.

The use of chemically crude reagents is probably a reflection of the fact that enzyme-labelled assays are not generally as sensitive as their radioisotope-labelled equivalents.

One useful feature of the enzyme-labelled immunoassay methods is the visual detection signal. Where only a qualitative result, either positive or negative, is required or even a semi-quantitative result, as with sample dilutions, the observation of the colour response can be made by eye, avoiding the use of any instrumentation altogether.

Further Reading

Engvall E. (1980). Enzyme immunoassay ELISA and EMIT. In: *Methods in Enzymology, Vol. 70: Immunochemical Techniques, Part A*. London: Academic Press.

O'Sullivan M.J., Marks V. (1981). Methods for the preparation of enzyme-antibody conjugates for use in enzyme immunoassay. In: *Methods in Enzymology, Vol. 73: Immunochemical Techniques, Part B*. London: Academic Press.

Various authors (1981). Immunoassay dependent on enzyme-labelled tracers. In: *Methods in Enzymology, Vol. 73: Immunochemical Techniques, Part B*. pp.471–577. London: Academic Press.

Voller A., Bidwell D. (1980). *The Enzyme Linked Immunosorbent Assay (ELISA)*, Vols. 1 & 2. Guernsey: MicroSystems Ltd.

CHAPTER SEVEN

Fluorescent-Labelled Immunoassay

Fluorescence

When a molecule absorbs radiation energy, electrons can be redistributed, giving rise to an excited state. For some molecules, the extra energy, instead of being lost to surrounding molecules, may be emitted as the electrons return to the ground state. This emitted radiation, in the form of light, is called fluorescence.

The excitation energy can be absorbed from photons of light at a particular wavelength. As some energy is usually lost before emission of radiation occurs, the emitted light has lower energy, and thus, a longer wavelength than the absorbed light.

The difference between the peak wavelengths of excitation and of fluorescence emission is called the Stokes shift (Figure 7.1). A large Stokes shift gives rise to better discrimination and more precise detection.

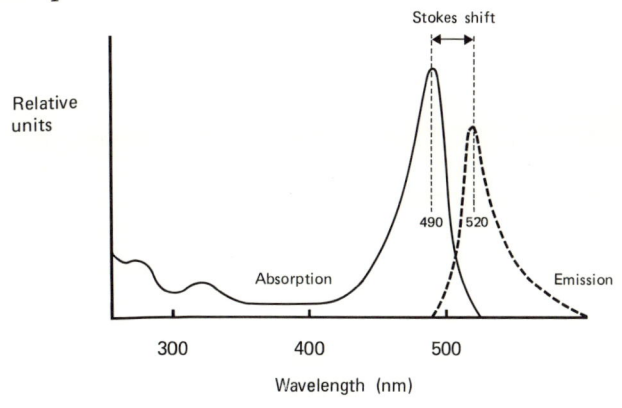

Figure 7.1 *Absorption and emission spectra for a fluorophore (fluorescein); the difference between the main peak of emitted fluorescence and the main peak of absorbed light is called the Stokes shift.*

Another important parameter of fluorescence is quantum efficiency, defined by the proportion of emitted fluorescence to the number of quanta of light absorbed. Again, as some energy is lost, quantum efficiency is less than 1. When the quantum efficiency approaches 1, it indicates maximum efficiency.

The use of Fluorophores as Labels

The practice of using fluorescent-labelled immunological reagents, starting with the publication of Coons in 1941, predates by a number of years many other labelling procedures, including the use of radioisotopes. However, their extensive application in immunoassay methods was not to happen for some years after the first radioimmunoassays.

Table 7.1
Classification of Fluoroimmunoassays

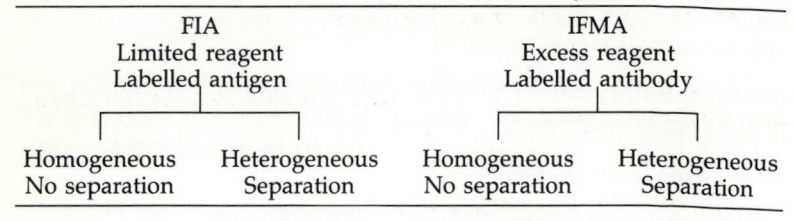

FIA		IFMA	
Limited reagent		Excess reagent	
Labelled antigen		Labelled antibody	
Homogeneous	Heterogeneous	Homogeneous	Heterogeneous
No separation	Separation	No separation	Separation

As with other labels, the use of fluorophores gives rise to a number of different immunoassay methods which can be divided into the basic categories of immunoassays, as considered in Table 7.1. Fundamentally, fluoroimmunoassays and immunofluorometric assays are identical to immunoassays using other labels, only limited or extended in sensitivity and precision by the constraints of particular fluorescence measurements. However, because of the susceptibility of fluorophores to modification by only minor changes in the molecular environment, fluorescent-labelled immunoassay methods are being found to be useful for development of homogeneous systems, i.e. an assay without a separation step. This characteristic of fluorescence, in itself a severe limitation of the method, has proved to be an

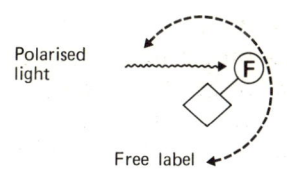

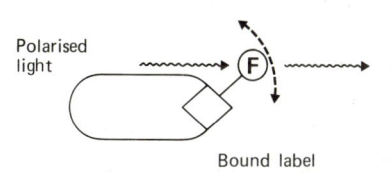

Figure 7.2 *Polarisation fluoroimmunoassay; a fluorophore, excited by plane polarised light, can emit polarised fluorescence. However, the rapid movement of a small fluorescent-labelled antigen reduces or eliminates the emission of plane polarised fluorescence. Following binding to the much larger antibody, movement is restricted, allowing for emission of plane polarised fluorescence. This can be used as a basis for a simple homogeneous immunoassay.*

advantage in terms of simplifying immunoassay procedures, providing sensitivity is not required.

Polarisation Fluoroimmunoassay

Polarised excitation light will give rise to fluorescence emission polarised in the same plane, providing the excited molecule does not shift its orientation in the time between excitation and emission. Although this time interval is usually very short (a few nanoseconds), small molecules will rotate sufficiently to reduce the quantity of fluorescence emission polarised in the original plane. Antibody bound antigen, on the other hand, constrained in its ability to rotate by the large molecular size of the antibody, will emit polarised fluorescence in the same plane as the excitation light. This phenomenon provides the basis of an interesting homogeneous fluoroimmunoassay (Figure 7.2) with its capacity to discriminate between antibody-bound antigen and free antigen without the need for physical separation.

Quenching and Enhancement Fluoroimmunoassays

In an analagous way to homogeneous enzyme immunoassays, fluorophores used in labelled antigens can give reduced (quenching) or increased (enhancement) fluorescence when bound by antibodies. Like the equivalent enzyme immunoassays, enhancement fluoroimmunoassays are not common. It is interesting to note that one antigen (thyroxine), for which a successful enhancement enzyme immunoassay was developed, also turns out to be suitable for assay by enhancement fluoroimmunoassay. The fluorophore, when coupled to the antigen thyroxine, has a low quantum efficiency, perhaps due to quenching effects of the iodine in the molecule. The quantum efficiency of the label increases considerably when the fluorophore labelled thyroxine is bound by the antibody (Figure 7.3). Maximum fluorescence in this system is achieved when most of the label is bound by antibody, i.e. in the absence of antigen. As the concentration of antigen increases, then less label will be bound by the limiting concentration of antibody and there will be a reduction in fluorescence.

Quenching fluoroimmunoassays are more common than enhancement assays. Fluorescence is not significantly im-

Free - impaired fluorescence

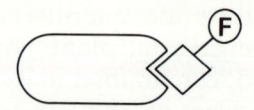

Bound - enhanced fluorescence

Figure 7.3 *Enhancement fluoroimmunoassay; a fluorophore when coupled to an antigen can show impaired fluorescence. The quenching effect of the antigen on the fluorophore can be removed by binding to antibody. This change in signal can be used as a basis for an homogeneous immunoassay.*

Free - fluorescence (unimpaired)

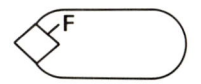

Bound - quenching of fluorescence

Figure 7.4 *Quenching fluoroimmunoassay; most fluorophores when coupled to antigens show no reduction in fluorescence. However, in some cases, the binding of antibody may reduce or quench the fluorescence.*

Anti - fluorophore

Free

Steric hindrance

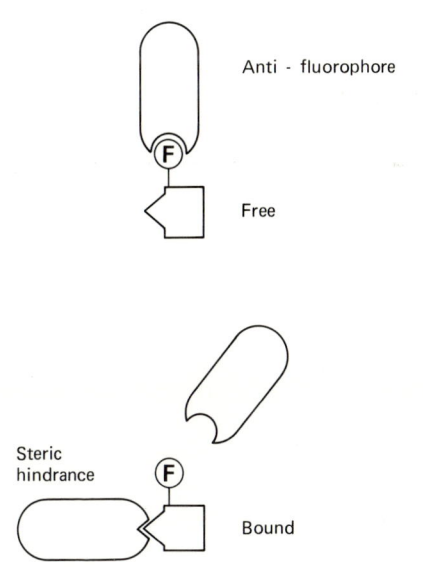

Bound

Figure 7.5 *Indirect quenching fluoroimmunoassay; the binding of a fluorophore by a specific antifluorophore antibody leads to quenching of the fluorescence. When the antigen–fluorophore conjugate is bound by the primary antibody, steric hindrance may prevent the antifluorophore from quenching the fluorescence. Increasing concentration of antigen leads to a greater proportion of labelled antigen in the free fraction and hence to increased quenching.*

paired when the fluorophore is coupled to antigens. For a few antibody–antigen reactions, binding of the antibody impairs, or quenches, the fluorescence of the label (Figure 7.4). Quenching, where it occurs, is not always a feature of all antibodies to a given hapten, and is also not applicable to the measurement of large molecule-like proteins. Maximum quenching occurs at zero unlabelled antigen concentration and decreases as the unlabelled antigen concentration increases. As quenching decreases, the fluorescence measured increases.

A novel innovation, indirect quenching, has made it possible to apply quenching principles to the measurement of large molecules (Figure 7.5). Indirect quenching employs a second antibody directed to the fluorophore. Binding of the antibody to the fluorophore quenches the fluorescence. However, when the large antigen labelled with fluorophores is bound to its own antibody, steric hindrance prevents the binding of the antifluorophore antibody and thus reduces the quenching effect. This technique is not usually applicable to small molecules (i.e. below about 20 000 molecular weight). The method is also known as fluorescence protection immunoassay (FPIA).

Antibodies that directly quench the fluorophore of a fluorescent-labelled hapten are not common. Quenching using the indirect quenching of FPIA is usually not applicable to small molecules. Alternative binding fluoroimmunoassay is an interesting development that allows indirect quenching principles to be applied to the assay of haptens and small molecules. The principle of alternative binding fluoroimmunoassay depends on a complex of the antihapten antibody and the antifluorophore antibody. In the absence of unlabelled hapten, this complex will be able to bind either end of the fluorescent-labelled hapten (Figure 7.6). As the concentration of unlabelled hapten increases progressively, more of the hapten binding sites become occupied, leaving only the fluorophore binding site available for binding of the fluorescent label. As more binding of the fluorescent label at the fluorophore end yields less fluorescence, increasing concentrations of hapten is measured by a quenching of fluorescence.

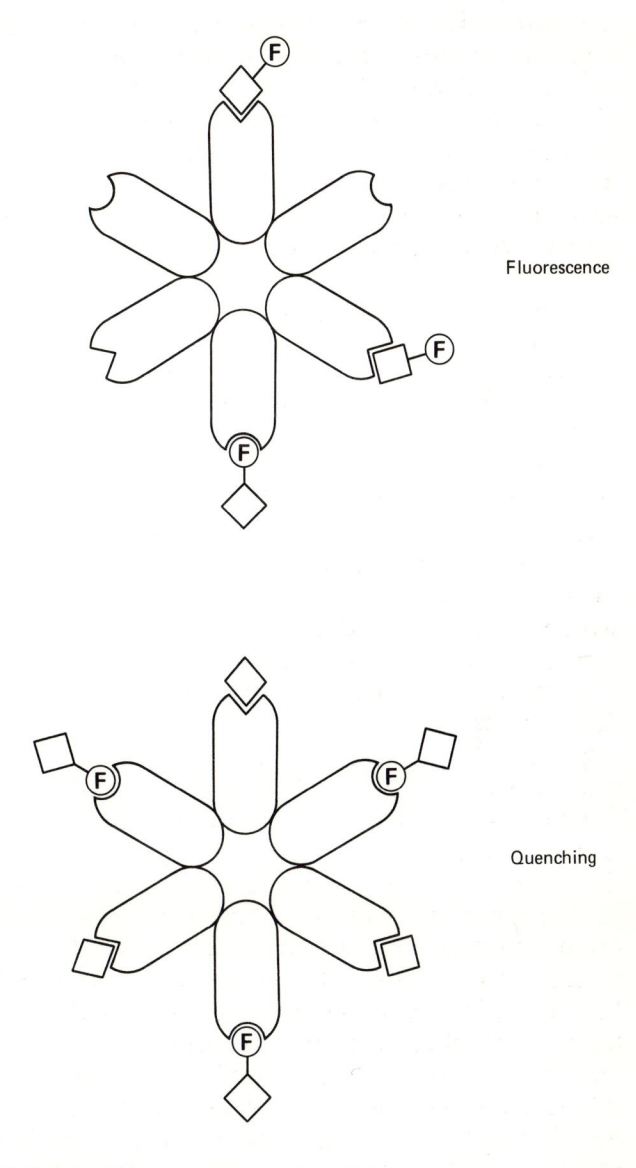

Figure 7.6 *Alternative binding fluoroimmunoassay; a complex of primary antibody and antifluorophore will bind an antigen–fluorophore conjugate at either end, yielding some fluorescence. With increasing concentrations of antigen, more conjugate will be bound at the fluorophore end, with the result of some quenching.*

Fluorescent Excitation Transfer Fluoroimmunoassay (FETI)

Different fluorophores usually have different absorption and emission spectra. However, the absorption peak of one fluorophore may overlap with the emission peak of another fluorophore. If the second fluorophore is placed in the immediate vicinity of the first, quenching of the fluorescent emission takes place through transfer of energy. This principle has been used in FETI by coupling one fluorophore to the antigen and the other fluorophore to the antibody. Binding of the antigen by the antibody leads to juxtaposition of both fluorophores and subsequent quenching (Figure 7.7).

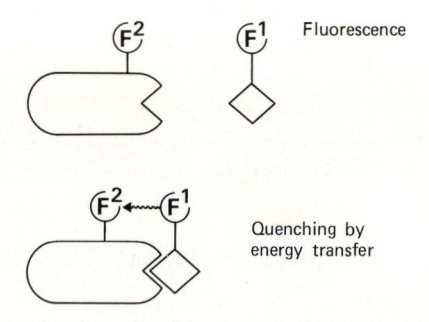

Figure 7.7 *Fluorescent excitation transfer fluoroimmunoassay; the juxtaposition of two different fluorophores, F^1 and F^2, can lead to quenching of fluorescence by energy transfer. The absorption spectrum of one fluorophore must overlap with the emission spectrum of the other fluorophore.*

Heterogeneous Fluoroimmunoassays

Despite the considerable advantage of an immunoassay without a separation step, homogeneous fluoroimmunoassays do have a number of limitations. Background fluorescence is often very high, particularly if biological samples are being used. Any one type of homogeneous fluoroimmunoassay seems to have limited application. The production of suitable reagents, particularly for quenching principles, is often technically complex and extemporaneous. Perhaps for these reasons, fluoroimmunoassays incorporating a separation step have generally proved more practical and have wider applications.

The principles of fluoroimmunoassay follow those outlined for immunoassays in general. The use of solid-phase reagents is perhaps much more a pre-requisite in fluoroimmunoassay than in many other types of immunoassays due to the nature of fluorescence. Fluorescence is readily changed or modified by minor changes in the molecular environment.

Antibodies coupled to a solid phase such as particles or beads are reacted with antigen and fluorescent label and then separated before fluorescent end-point detection. Fluorescence in the supernatant (free fraction) can be measured in tubes with the precipitated antibody-bound fraction *'in situ'*. To improve precision and sensitivity, the supernatant is removed and the precipitated fraction is extensively washed. Fluorescence of the bound fraction is then measured following resuspension of the precipitate or following elution of the label.

Immunofluorometric Assays (IFMA)

Assays using the immunometric principle, i.e. excess antibody reagent, and with the label attached to the antibody, have been developed for use with fluorescent labels. In general, these follow the principle illustrated for the IRMA and the ELISA. Separation is achieved using solid-phase antibody or solid-phase antigen, again directly analogous to the basic IRMA or ELISA. The IFMA is usually not as sensitive as ELISA and, almost invariably, not as sensitive as IRMA. However, some recent modifications and developments may lead ultimately to improved performance with immunofluorometric assays and thus to more widespread application.

Homogeneous IFMA

Using the same principle of fluorescence excitation transfer used in FETI, it is possible to apply IFMA without a

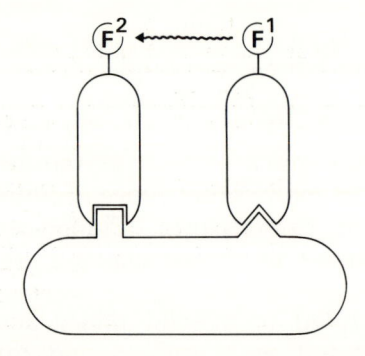

Figure 7.8 *Fluorescent excitation transfer fluoroimmunoassay for large molecules; two species of antibodies reacting with different antigenic sites on a single large molecule, such as a protein, are labelled with different fluorophores. In the presence of the antigen, binding of both antibodies leads to juxtaposition of the fluorophores and subsequent quenching by energy transfer (see Figure 7.7).*

separation step to the measurement of large antigens, such as proteins. Two populations of antibody are labelled with two different fluorophores, overlapping in their respective absorption and emission peaks (see p. 87). One molecule of antigen, being of sufficient size and with several antigenic binding sites, may bind both antibodies labelled with their respective different fluorophores. Coincidence of the two fluorophores gives rise to energy transfer between the two, with a subsequent quenching or reduction of fluorescence (Figure 7.8). Although this technique has limited sensitivity, it does have the considerable advantage of non-separation assays.

Choice of Fluorophores

The main types of fluorophore used currently as labels in immunoassay are listed in Table 7.2, together with some relevant features.

Fluorescein is a very satisfactory fluorophore in many respects and has been very extensively used. One of its main advantages is that it is readily available in an activated form for direct coupling to the antigen or antibody. Both the isocyanate or the isothiocyanate forms of fluorescein are

Table 7.2
Fluorophores used on Labels

Fluorophore	Stokes shift	Features
Fluorescein (isothiocyanate)	492–518 nm (26 nm)	Chemically stable Quantum yields—approx. 90% Fluorescence lifetime—5 nsec
Rhodamine (isothiocyanate)	550–585 nm (35 nm)	Quantum yield—approx. 70% Fluorescence lifetime—3 nsec
Umbelliferone	380–450 nm (70 nm)	Chemically stable
Lanthanide chelates	e.g. 330–613 nm (>270 nm)	Narrow emission band Fluorescence lifetime 10–1000 μsec Quantum yield usually low

reactive and have been used. Fluorescein isothiocyanate is the reagent of choice, and coupling to antigens is very readily and simply achieved as the protocol in Table 7.3 illustrates.

Both fluorescein and rhodamines show good chemical stability and, in practice, as labels, have a well proven record. As the spectra of fluorescein and rhodamine overlap, these two fluorophores have been used for fluorescence excitation transfer in both immunoassay and immunometric versions.

Both fluorescein and rhodamines have relatively small Stokes shift which limits the methodology in some respects. Interference can arise in fluorescent measurements from light scattering, but these problems can be generally resolved by discriminating instrumentation.

Both umbelliferones and lanthanide chelates have larger Stokes shifts, but their use as labels in immunoassays is relatively recent and they are still untried in many respects. The lanthanide chelates have the potential of ideal

Table 7.3
Preparation of Fluorescein Conjugate

1. Approximately 10 μmole antigen (with amine group)
2. Add 500 μl carbonate buffer (pH 9·0, 0·05M) at 4°C
3. Slowly add 500 μl fluorescein isothiocyanate (10 mg/ml) in carbonate buffer (pH 9·0, 0·05M) at 4°C
4. Stir overnight at 4°C
5. Purify products

NB. Can use methanol (+0·1% triethylamine) as alternative solvent system.

fluorophores, but the coupling between fluorophore and antigen has presented some problems and the fluorophore can be labile, seriously restricting use for labels. This situation is being resolved and a few assays have recently been published in which lanthanide chelates have been used as labels. One very interesting aspect of the fluorescence of the lanthanide chelates is the very long fluorescence lifetime. The fluorescence lifetime is the time taken for the fluorescence to disappear when no further excitation energy is available. The fluorescence lifetime of the lanthanide chelate fluorophores is of the order of 100 microseconds, compared to 5 nanoseconds for fluoroscein. This feature has led to the possibility of using time-resolved fluorimetry to improve the performance of fluorescent immunoassay methods.

Time Resolved Fluorimetry

Background fluorescence is one of the main problems with the use of fluorescence, and its presence can severely limit practical use of fluorescent immunoassay methods. However, background fluorescence present in most biological material has the relatively short lifetime of a few nanoseconds. For fluorophores with long fluorescence lifetimes, it is possible to measure fluorescence at a time when virtually all the background fluorescence has disappeared (Figure 7.9). Although the specific fluorescence itself may also be less, the signal-to-noise ratio will be much higher. The signal-to-noise ratio is the most significant aspect for improving the precision and sensitivity of detection.

For time-resolved fluorimetry the sample is excited with a short pulse of light and not the continuous beam of light in the conventional fluorimeter. All fluorophores, including those non-specific fluorophores responsible for the background, reach an excited state and then give rise to fluorescent emission. For lanthanide chelates, the lanthanide or rare earth element is responsible for energy absorption, which is then translocated to the chelating molecule, and subsequently yields a fluorescent emission characteristic of the chelates.

Another useful feature of the fluorescent characteristics of

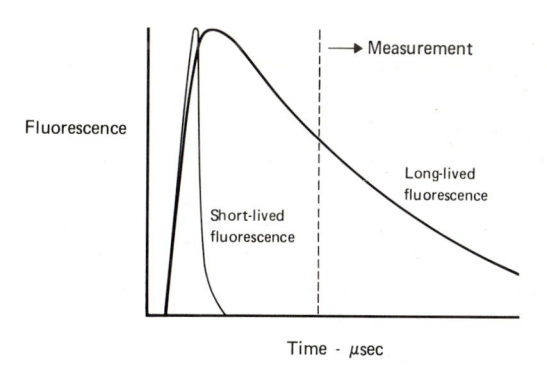

Figure 7.9 *Time-resolved fluorescence; measurement after a certain time avoids interference from short-lived background fluorescence.*

the lanthanide chelates is the very sharp and narrow emission spectra, which improves discrimination providing appropriate instrumentation is available. The addition of laser light, with the attendant advantages of high intensity, monochromaticity and ease of collimation to the instruments used for time-resolved fluorimetry, may improve further fluorescent measurements.

Further Reading

Rhys Williams A.T. (1980). *Fluoroimmunoassay: A Review of Present Methods.* Perkin-Elmer Limited.

Smith D.S., Al-Hakiem M.H.H., Landon J. (1981). A review of fluoroimmunoassay and immunofluorometric assay. *Ann. Clin. Biochem;* **18**: 253–74.

Various authors. (1981). Fluorescence immunoassay methods. In: *Methods in enzymology, Vol. 74. Immunochemical Techniques, Part C.* London: Academic Press.

CHAPTER EIGHT

Luminescent-Labelled Immunoassays

Luminescence

Luminescence is a very similar phenomenon to fluorescence. Whereas the exciting energy in fluorescence is in the form of light, in luminescence it is provided by a chemical reaction.

Luminescence can be divided into two general types, namely chemiluminescence and bioluminescence reactions. A bioluminescent reaction is one essentially derived from a living organism; for example, the well-known firefly luciferase system. The light-producing reaction is directed by specific enzymes. Bioluminescent reactions are widely distributed within the animal and plant kingdoms, especially in ocean-dwelling species. Bioluminescent materials are available in useful amounts from certain bacteria and fungi. Chemiluminescent reactions produce light from simple chemical reactions, involving action of oxygen or a peroxide on certain oxidation organic substrates. After excitation of the luminescent substrate, some of the molecules emit the energy in the form of light, whilst others lose the energy in the form of heat. The relative proportion of emitted light (the photon efficiency), is a useful measure of the efficiency of reactions. Bioluminescent reactions usually have photon efficiencies of between 10 and 90%, whilst chemiluminescent reactions often have photon efficiencies of about 1%. An important development in recent years has been the enhancement of chemiluminescent reactions to give much higher photon efficiencies.

Luminescent Reactions

There are two main types of bioluminescent reactions, the firefly luciferase system and the bacterial luciferase system

FIREFLY BIOLUMINESCENCE

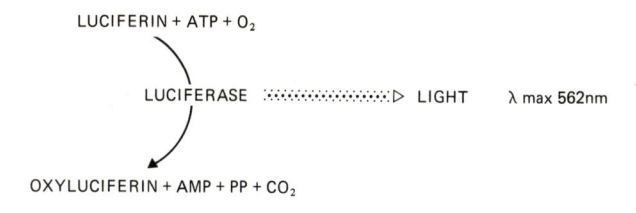

LUCIFERIN + ATP + O_2

⟶ LUCIFERASE ⟶ LIGHT λ max 562nm

OXYLUCIFERIN + AMP + PP + CO_2

BACTERIAL BIOLUMINESCENCE

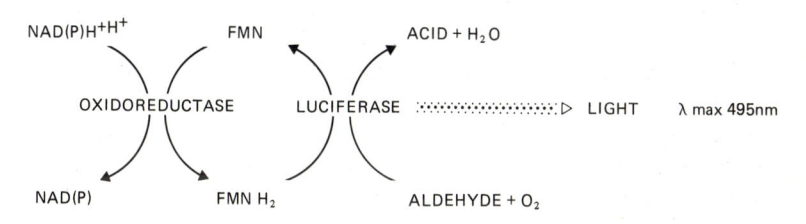

$NAD(P)H + H^+$ FMN   ACID + H_2O

OXIDOREDUCTASE   LUCIFERASE ⟶ LIGHT λ max 495nm

NAD(P) $FMN H_2$ ALDEHYDE + O_2

Figure 8.1 *The two types of bioluminescent reactions.*

(Figure 8.1). The purified firefly luciferase system is specific for ATP, with a photon being produced for almost every molecule of ATP reacted. The other luciferase enzymes, such as bacterial, are specific for either NADH or NADPH, but they have a much lower photon efficiency (about 10%) than that found for the firefly enzyme. Because the firefly luciferase system has a greater photon efficiency than the bacterial luciferase system, it is potentially more sensitive as an analytical technique.

The main chemiluminescent reaction studied (Figure 8.2) is the production of light from luminol in the presence of peroxides. The photon efficiency is about 1%. The reaction requires a catalyst, certain metals or haemins, and an alkaline pH.

Luminol chemiluminescence can also be catalysed by a peroxidase at neutral pH. The reaction kinetics of luminescent reactions vary from fast to slow depending on a number

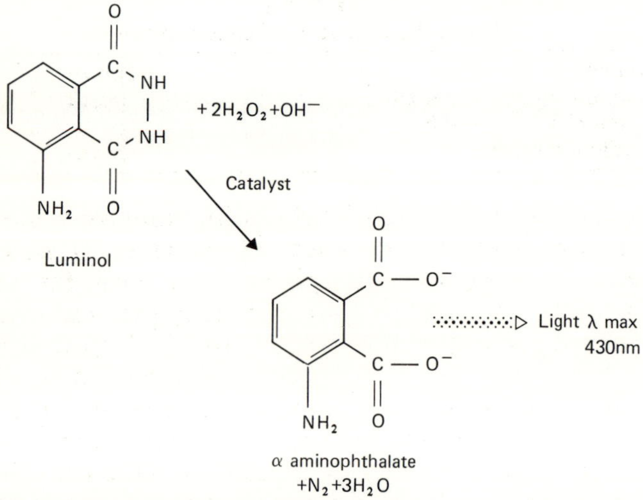

Figure 8.2 *Chemiluminescent reaction of luminol.*

of factors, such as the concentration of rate-limiting substances. The light emitted from fast reaction kinetics, e.g. luminol chemiluminescence, can be measured as the maximum intensity of a single pulse. Where the light is emitted continuously, the measurement can be made over a preset time or as a continuous signal.

Application of Luminescence to Immunoassays

The use of luminescence in chemical and biochemical analyses is relatively new and in many ways the subject is still in a developmental stage. However, the considerable interest shown in the technique indicates that luminometry could be a major analytical method in many disciplines.

With respect to the novel application of luminometry to immunoassay methods, there have been relatively few reports of luminescent-labelled assays in comparison with those using other types of label. Because of the high sensitivity (Table 8.1) inherent in the technique, and the potential simplicity of the instrumentation, the application of luminescent labels in immunoassay methods should increase dramatically.

Table 8.1
Potential Sensitivity of Luminescence

Luminol	approx. 10^{-15} mol
Bioluminescence (bacterial)	approx. 10^{-17} mol
Bioluminescence (firefly)	approx. 10^{-18} mol
Acridinium ester	approx. 10^{-18} mol

The use of luminescent labels in immunoassay methods conforms broadly to the variety of examples given in the previous chapter for fluorophores. As with fluorescent labels, solid-phase reagents are extremely practical in allowing the easy removal of interference from biological samples. Also, there have been early reports of homogeneous luminescent immunoassays. At present, these do not appear to be as successful as the fluorescent-labelled ones. As the subject is still in its infancy, it is more useful to consider the potential ways that luminescence can be used to monitor or label immunological reagents rather than detail types of luminescent immunoassays.

The Use of Chemiluminescence

The simplest and most direct way of using luminescence for monitoring immunoassays or immunometric assays is by coupling the luminescent material, e.g. luminol, to the antigen or antibody. A number of chemiluminescent substrates are available (see Table 8.2), but most use has been made of the isoluminol derivatives and the acridinium esters. The coupling of luminol to various antigens and proteins does not lead to very efficient luminescent labels. This may be partly explained by the low solubility of

Table 8.2
Chemiluminescent Substrates

Luminol
Isoluminol
Pyrogallol
Protohaemin (catalyst)
Aminobutylethyl-n-isoluminol (ABEI)
Aminohexylethyl-n-ethyl-isoluminol (AHEI)
Acridinium esters

luminol. Also, the luminol derivatives may have considerably reduced luminescent activity, perhaps from steric hindrances due to the position of the reactive amine group.

Isoluminol and its Derivatives

Isoluminol can be used to couple to immunological reagents through a reactive amino group (-NH$_2$). This reactive group can be coupled directly to antibodies or antigens using a simple coupling reagent, e.g. carbodiimide. Unlike luminol, coupled isoluminol does not usually lose luminescent activity and may even exhibit increased activity. The main problem with the use of isoluminol, like luminol, is its low solubility. Isoluminol has lower solubility than luminol, and this generally leads to inferior performance when it is used to label reagents.

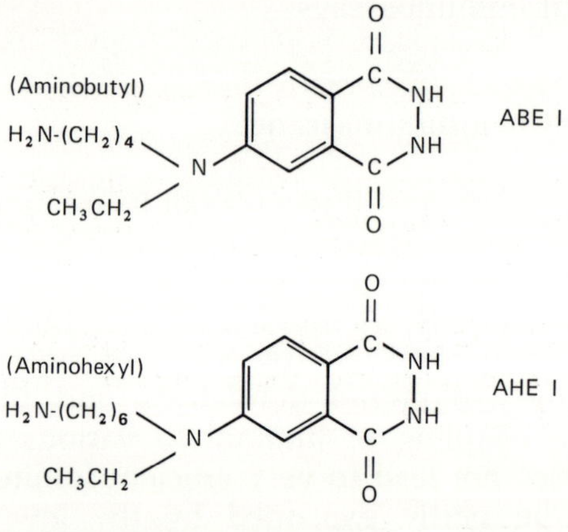

Figure 8.3 *Two derivatives of isoluminol; aminobutyl*-n-*ethyl-isoluminol (ABEI), and aminohexyl*-n-*ethyl-isoluminol (AHEI).*

The two common derivatives of isoluminol, aminobutyl-*n*-ethyl-isoluminol (ABEI) and aminohexyl-*n*-ethyl-isoluminol (AHEI), have much better solubility characteristics than luminol or isoluminol, thus resolving one of the problems. The structure of ABEI and AHEI vary only in the length of the side chain (Figure 8.3). The light yield is greatest from

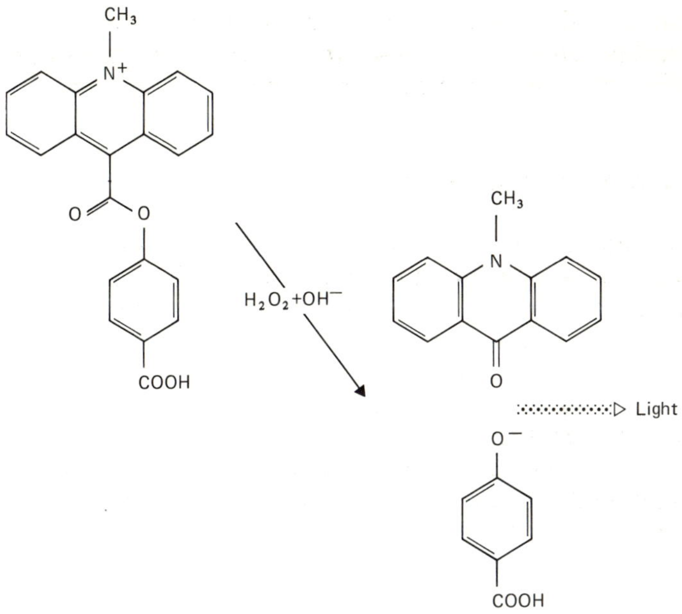

Figure 8.4 *Chemiluminescent reaction of acridinium esters.*

AHEI (side chain, $n = 6$) compared to ABEI (side chain, $n = 4$). However, the aminobutyl derivative is least sensitive to variations in the time interval before addition of oxidation reagents.

Both ABEI and AHEI are available commercially as pure reagents. For general use, the aminobutyl derivative seems the most satisfactory.

Use of Acridinium Esters

Acridinium esters (see Figure 8.4), are more luminescent than luminol and can be used as chemiluminescent labels to give assays with enhanced sensitivity. Analogous to the use of luminol or isoluminol derivatives, they are coupled directly to the immunological reagent, that is either the antigen or the antibody. They can then be used as luminescent labels in either a luminescent immunoassay (LIA) or an immunoluminometric assay (ILMA). Because the acridinium esters have a potential light yield up to a hundred times that of luminol, their use as labels in immunoassay methods can mean a corresponding increase in sensitivity. An additional advantage is the lack of a quenching effect when further molecules are coupled to the reagent. The most active conjugates are reported to give almost 10^{19} counts per molecule of conjugate. This means that immunoassay methods using these labels are theoretically capable of achieving better sensitivities than the corresponding radiolabelled ones.

Peroxidase-Labelled Conjugates

The peroxidase enzyme can also be used for labelling immunological reagents (as in Figure 8.5). The peroxidase, a catalyst in luminol chemiluminescence, is monitored in one of the several chemiluminescent reactions. This particular variant benefits from the wide availability of peroxidase conjugates, many of which are available commercially. It has

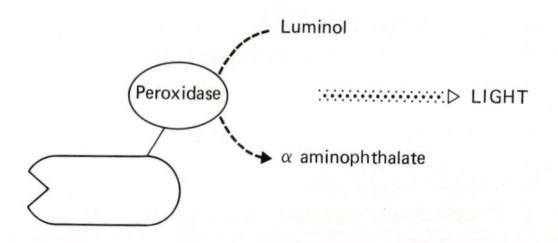

Figure 8.5 *The use of peroxidase enzyme as a chemiluminescent label; the peroxidase enzyme catalyses the luminescent reaction of luminol.*

also been designated the luminescent enzyme immunoassay (LEIA). One advantage of the use of this particular catalyst as a label over other catalysts of luminescent reactions is that it is less prone to a loss of activity when incorporated into conjugates. The peroxidase catalysed oxidation of luminol can be enhanced by the addition to the reaction medium of synthetic luciferin, a component of firefly bioluminescence. This enhanced luminescent reaction can be used to give immunoassays with much lower levels of detection.

The Use of Bioluminescence

Bioluminescence suffers from the relative scarcity of reagents and, as a consequence, a concomitant increase in expense. Although the firefly luciferase system has the highest photon yield, other bioluminescent reagents derived from bacteria, fungi or the earthworm are likely to be available in greater amounts. The firefly bioluminescent reaction, should give the most sensitive immunological reagents, but where maximum sensitivity is not the dominant factor, other factors, such as availability and cost, will be more important.

In principle, any of the components of bioluminescent reactions could be used as labels in immunoassay methods. Candidates for forming bioluminescent conjugate labels are listed in Table 8.3.

Table 8.3
Candidates for Bioluminescent Labels

Firefly System
  Luciferase
  Luciferin
  Adenosine triphosphate (ATP)

Bacterial System
  Luciferase
  Nicotinamide adenine dinucleotide (NAD)
  Flavin mononucleotide (FMN)
  Oxidoreductases

The luciferase enzymes, either firefly or bacterial, and the specific oxidoreductases, are very easily conjugated to antigens or antibodies. However, a significant loss of enzyme activity often results in the case of the luciferases. The use of luciferase as bioluminescent labels does not seem to be a practical proposition.

Covalent coupling of any one of the cofactors such as ATP, FMN or NAD is possible. However, the conjugated cofactor may well lose some reactivity with the very specific luciferase enzyme. NAD has been used with some success and ATP is active, providing it is enzymatically released from the conjugate before measurement.

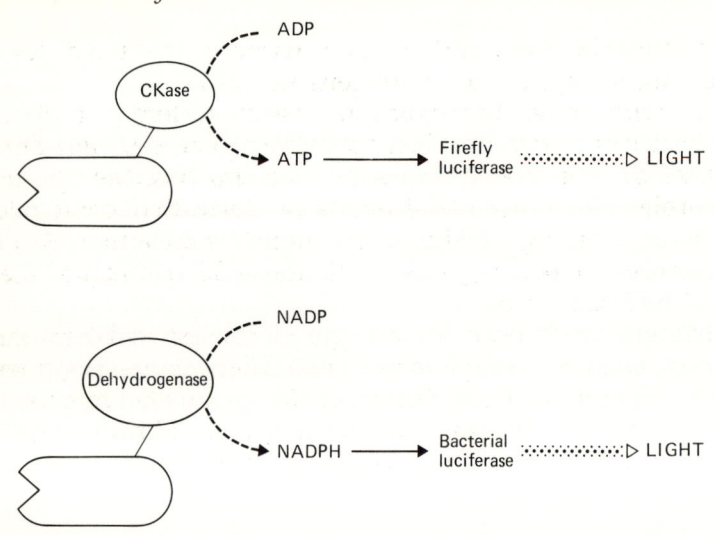

Figure 8.6 *Enzymes as bioluminescent labels; both creatine kinase (CKase) and glucose-6-phosphate dehydrogenase can be used as labels as their products are substrates for bioluminescent reactions.*

An alternative to these specific components as labels, is the use of non-specific enzymes that can link directly into the bioluminescence reaction. Two such possibilities are illustrated in Figure 8.6. Both creatine kinase and dehydrogenase enzymes are readily available. Glucose-6-phosphate dehydrogenase is used to reduce NADP and malate dehydrogenase is used to reduce NAD. The dehydrogenase enzyme conjugates are commonly used in enzyme immunoassay methods and are widely available.

The use of dehydrogenase conjugates represents a very practical approach to realising the potential of monitoring with bioluminescence.

Homogeneous Luminescent Immunoassays

Analogous to the use of the fluorophores as labels, the light yield from luminescence-labelled conjugates can be affected by binding with the antibody. As a consequence, it is possible to discriminate between the antibody-bound fraction and the unbound antigen without the need for a separation step, i.e. an homogeneous assay.

As with other homogeneous assay systems, antibody binding can lead to a reduction in the signal, i.e. quenching assays, or an increase in the signal, i.e. enhanced assays. For example, some antigen–isoluminol derivative conjugates give enhanced light yields when bound by the antibody, the enhancement being greater with the ABEI conjugate than the AHEI conjugate.

The colour or peak wavelength of the emitted light can also be altered through antibody binding. At present, there are no reports using a change in this parameter to give an homogeneous luminescent immunoassay. However, it is reasonable to expect these to appear soon.

Salient Features of Luminescent Immunoassay

Although luminescence has the potential to compete with radiolabel for maximum sensitivity, it is a detection system prone to interference.

Variations in both pH and temperature can have critical effects on luminescence. Not only can a change in pH reduce quantum yield, but it can shift the light emission spectrum leading to a change in maximum wavelength.

Turbidity of the reaction is not usually a problem in luminescence detection, as most luminometers are designed to monitor the total light emitted, and are not limited to measurements in one direction.

Over the years, some interference in the bioluminescent luciferase reactions has resulted from impurities in the reagent preparations themselves. However, the present batches of commercial reagents have resolved this problem with highly purified preparations.

Endogenous nucleotides and nucleotide-converting enzymes in biological samples can often interfere in those reactions where the concentrations of the nucleotides, NAD(P)H and ATP, are critical. In common with all enzyme-related reactions, the luminescent enzyme system will also be susceptible to the possibility of interference from endogenous enzyme substrates and enzyme inhibitors. The luciferase enzymes are inhibited by high ionic strength, especially anions such as acetate and chloride.

More general interference can result from the effect of fluorescent lights on impurities in cuvettes or plastic tubes, and from minute amounts of impurities in the water. This last effect introduces a requirement for maximally purified water supplies.

The prevalence of potential interfering factors in luminescent reactions will, without doubt, predispose the technique to applications with solid-phase separation systems, particularly where sensitivity and specificity are issues. The luminescent label should be removed from the reaction mixture and washed to remove any interfering material, before the luminescence is measured. This removal and washing is most readily achieved with solid-phase reagents.

Although the application of luminescent labels to immunoassay methods represents a very small proportion of all immunoassay techniques at present, it should increase over the next few years. Luminometry may grow to play a dominant role in immunoassay methods because of its extreme sensitivity and potential widespread use.

Further Reading

Collins W.P., Barnard G.J., Kim J.B., Weerasekera D.A., Kohen F., Eshhar Z., Lindner H.R. (1983). Chemiluminescence immunoassay for plasma steroids and urinary steroid metabolites. In: *Immunoassays for Clinical Chemistry.* (Hunter W.M., Corrie J.E.T., eds.) Ch. 9, pp.373–97. Edinburgh: Churchill Livingstone.

Olsson T., Thore A. (1981). Chemiluminescence and its use in immunoassay. In: *Immunoassays for the 80s.* (Voller A., Bartlett A., Bidwell D., eds.) Ch. 9, pp.113–25. Lancaster: MTP Press.

CHAPTER NINE

Immunoprecipitation Assays

Precipitation

Mixing an antigen with an antiserum can give rise to a visible precipitate. This fact, one of the earliest known aspects of antigen–antibody reactions, was noted by Krause in 1897. The primary reaction of one molecule of an antigen with one molecule of an antibody does not give rise to precipitation. A secondary reaction seems to be necessary for the formation of a visible precipitate. Cross-linking between multivalent antigens and antibodies seems to be the most likely basis of this secondary reaction. Mixtures of antigen and antibody that are likely to be soluble are listed in Table 9.1. Immunoprecipitation seems to depend on the formation of multivalent complexes of at least a greater complexity than those listed.

Table 9.1
Soluble Complexes

Antibody	Antigen
1	1
1	2
2	3

The Precipitin Test

Immunoprecipitation was the basis of one of the very earliest immunoassays, the precipitin test. The precipitin test of Heidelberger and Kendall in 1929 and 1935 (quantitative tests for antigens and antibodies), pre-dated the more sensitive immunoassays by several decades. In principle, a constant amount of antibody is reacted with varying concentrations of antigen. The immunoprecipitate is formed and removed by centrifugation. The protein content of the

112 Immunoassay

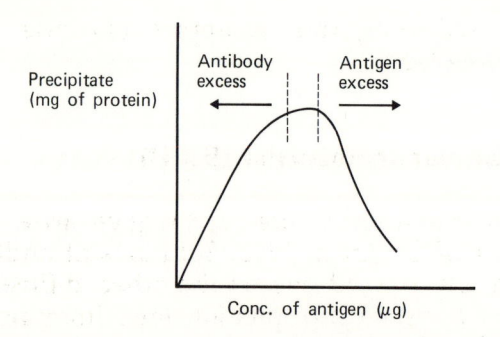

Figure 9.1 *The precipitin curve; in the precipitin test the amount of precipitate formed varies in relationship to the concentration of antigen. Maximum precipitation takes place when neither antibody nor antigen are in excess, i.e. at the point of equivalence. The biphasic response of this test, first published in 1929, indicates the principles of both the immunoassay (limited reagent) and the immunometric assay (excess reagent).*

precipitate is assayed by optical density or nitrogen determination (micro-Kjeldahl). The relationship between protein content of the precipitate and increasing concentrations of antigen gives a curve (Figure 9.1) from which it is possible to interpolate concentrations of antigen. The biphasic relationship is interesting in that it is a composite of the essential features of the two main categories of immunoassay methods already designated. The descending part of the curve, due to excess antigen, predicts the behaviour of the immunoassay with a limiting concentration of antibody. The ascending part of the curve, with excess antibody, predicts the behaviour of the immunometric assay.

The peak of the curve relates to maximum precipitation occurring at equivalence. It is this point of equivalence that is essentially the relevant end-point of immunoprecipitation techniques. This being so, immunoprecipitation techniques are not to be classified in either of the two categories already mentioned, but constitute a third category of immunoassay methods.

In this third category of methods, the antibodies and/or the antigens, migrate to form a visible precipitation line at a point of equivalence, in terms of concentration. The migration either takes place by diffusion or in an electrophoretic field. Although there are many varieties of these assays, the following four examples illustrate the basic procedures involved.

Single Radial Immunodiffusion (SRID)

The various immunodiffusion techniques arise from the original work of Oudin in 1948. Solutions of antibody and antigen carefully layered one on the other, diffuse in a test tube to form a visible precipitation line. Immunodiffusion now takes place in a more precise manner in gels (usually a simple agarose gel). The technique of single radial immunodiffusion was first described by Feinberg in 1957, and later versions by Mancini in 1965.

An agarose gel containing an even distribution of antibody is cast. This gel contains a number of wells, either cast or cut out. Various concentrations of antigen are introduced into the empty wells and allowed to diffuse into the gel. Diffusion continues until a discrete precipitation line appears. As this precipitation line should occur at the point of equivalence, the distance the line occurs from the well is proportional to the concentration of antigen (Figure 9.2). A gel containing the antigen can be used as an assay for antibodies.

Double Immunodiffusion (DID)

The double immunodiffusion technique, based on the work of Ouchterlony (1958), uses a plain gel containing neither antibody or antigen. Wells are either cast in the gel or punched out from the gel, and are usually arranged in a regular pattern around a central well (Figure 9.3). A suitable dilution of an antiserum is introduced into the central well and various antigens at varying concentrations are introduced into the surrounding wells. The position and shape of the resulting precipitation lines give information on the approximate concentrations of the antigens and on a variety of antigenic binding sites. The distance of lines from the antigen wells is an indication of concentration. Continuity of the line from adjacent wells indicates a common antigenic

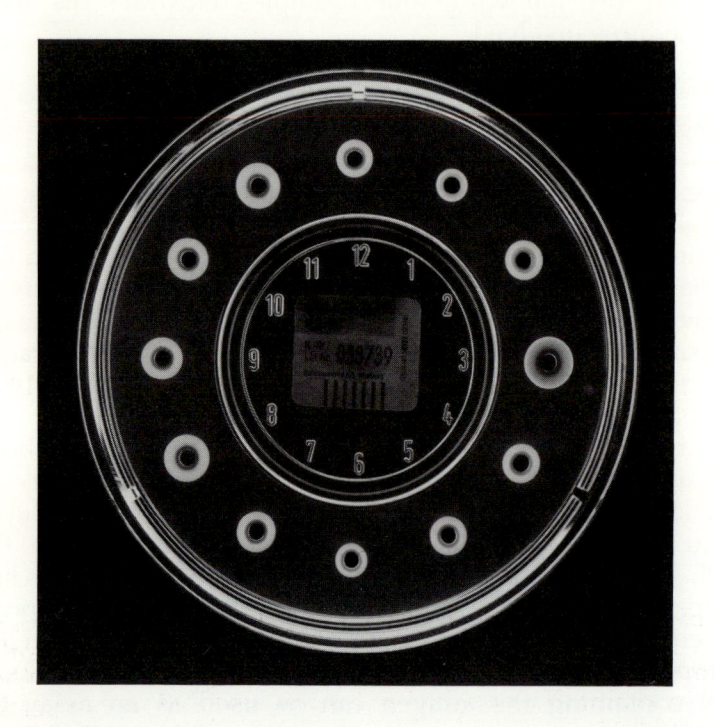

Figure 9.2 *Single radial immunodiffusion; antigen from the wells diffuse into a gel containing specific antibody. A precipitin line is formed at a distance from the well in proportion to the concentration of antigen. The diameter of the circular precipitation line gives a measure of the concentration of antigen. In this example, samples (wells 4–12) are assayed for human IgG by comparison with standards (wells 1–3).*

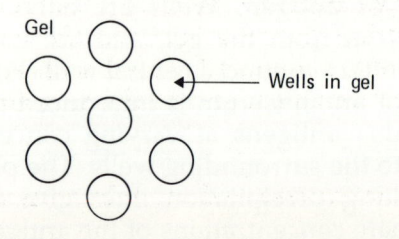

Figure 9.3 *Pattern of wells for double immunodiffusion; the central well is used for the antiserum, and the surrounding wells used for different antigens, or vice versa.*

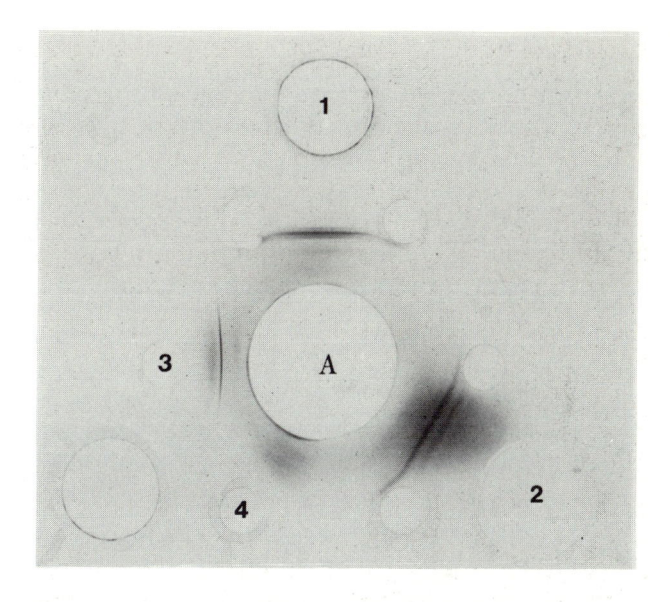

Figure 9.4 *Double immunodiffusion—Ouchterlony technique. Antigens diffuse from peripheral wells into the gel, where an immunoprecipitate is formed by reaction with the antiserum, which has diffused into the gel from the central well. In this example, the central well A contained sheep antiserum to* Candida albicans *somatic antigens. Wells 1 and 2 contained* C. albicans *somatic antigen at a concentration of 20 mg/ml. Well 3 contained* C. albicans *somatic antigen at a concentration of 2 mg/ml. Well 4 contained* Candida parapsilosis *somatic antigen at a concentration of 2 mg/ml.* NB: *Several precipitin lines can be seen because the antiserum was raised against a mixed antigen. (Gel by courtesy of James Carney, Mercia Diagnostics.)*

binding site, while crossing and spurs indicate the presence of different antigenic binding sites. A developed Ouchterlony plate in Figure 9.4 illustrates these various features. The Ouchterlony plate can be used with antigen in the central well and various antisera in the surrounding wells.

Electroimmunoassay—Rocket Immunoelectrophoresis

The assay by migration of antigens, in an electrophoretic field, into a gel containing antibody is the basis of electroimmunodiffusion, or as it is sometimes called, electroimmunoassay. The technique first described by Laurell in 1966 also goes under the name of rocket immunoelectrophoresis, or the Laurell rocket assay.

Agarose containing an antibody is poured to give a gel of uniform thickness. Wells are punched out of the gel at one end into which various samples are introduced. Electrophoresis is caried out, during which time the various samples migrate into the gel and form precipitation lines at the point of equivalence. The precipitation line for each sample has a characteristic rocket shape (Figure 9.5) and the

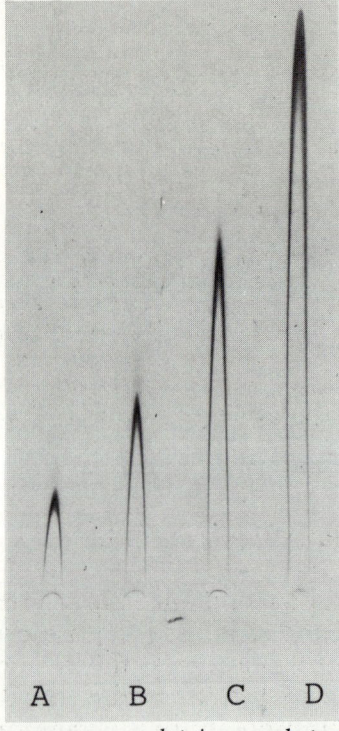

Figure 9.5 *Electroimmunoassay—rocket immunoelectrophoresis. Antigens migrate in an electric field into a gel containing antiserum. Immunoprecipitation occurs as a result of the reaction between specific antibody and antigen at a position of equivalence. The precipitin line describes the characteristic shape of a 'rocket'. The height of the 'rocket' is proportional to the concentration of antigen in the well. In this example, increasing concentrations of fragment E:A, 12·5 µg/ml; B, 25 µg/ml; C, 50 µg/ml; D, 100 µg/ml; were electrophoresised into a gel containing anti-human fibrogen fragment E. (Gel by courtesy of James Carnay, Mercia Diagnostics.)*

height of the rocket is proportional to the concentration of antigen. The greater concentration of antigen will migrate further into the gel before reaching a point of equivalence. The technique can be used successfully to quantitate two different antigens at the same time if run in a gel containing two specific antisera and if the respective rockets differ in shape or electrophoretic direction, i.e. one moves towards the cathode and one moves towards the anode.

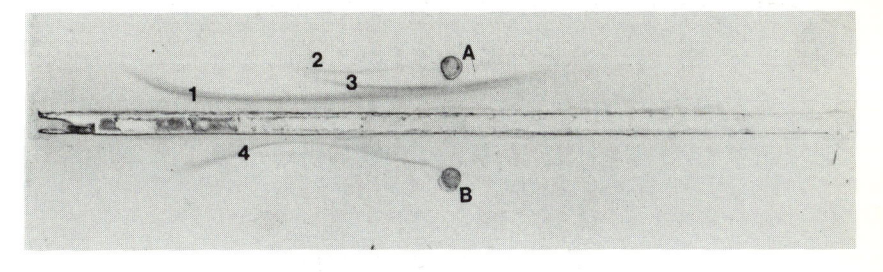

Figure 9.6 *Immunoelectrophoresis; components in a sample separate in an electric field. Following electrophoresis, an antiserum is placed in the trough and diffuses into the gel. In the gel, the antibodies react with various antigens giving precipitin lines. In this example, two serum samples are placed in wells (normal serum in Well A, serum from patient with myeloma in well B), and electrophoresised. Antihuman immunoglobulin antiserum is placed in the central trough. The labelled precipitin arcs indicate: 1, IgG; 2, IgA; 3, IgM; 4, myeloma protein. (Gel by courtesy of Frank Hay.)*

Crossed Immunoelectrophoresis

The more conventional immunoelectrophoresis is carried out as shown in Figure 9.6. Antigens are separated by electrophoresis into various components which then diffuse against an antibody migrating by diffusion from a trough cut alongside the electrophoretic run. This technique is used as a qualitative test to investigate the composition of crude antigens or mixtures. The extension of this technique into a second dimension improves the resolution of complex mixtures and adds a quantitative measure. A sample is separated by electrophoresis in one dimension and then migrates in a second dimension, again by electrophoresis, into an antibody-containing gel. As the various components migrate

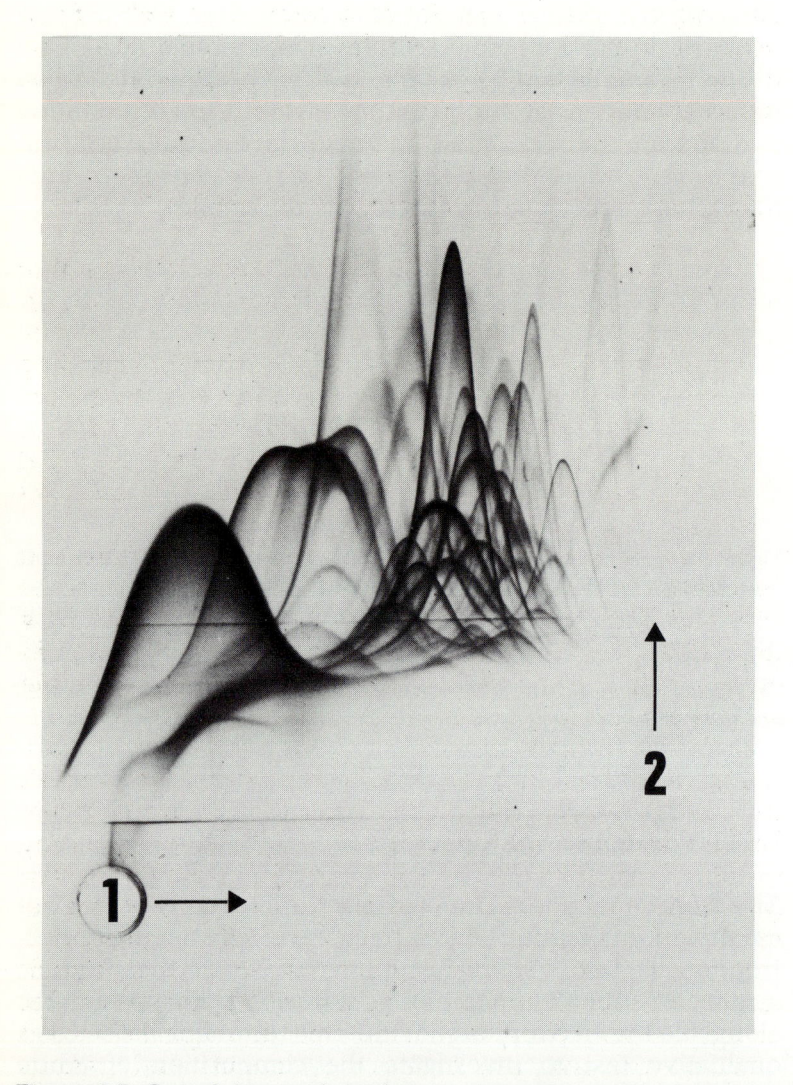

Figure 9.7 Crossed immunoelectrophoresis. A complex antigen mixture is separated by electrophoresis in one dimension (→1). Then electrophoresis is carried out across the gel into a second gel containing a polyvalent antiserum (→2). Distinct antigenic components give rise to the different arcs of precipitation. This figure shows crossed immunoelectrophoresis of a crude antigen mixture (at least 50 components) from a particular mycobacterium.
(Photograph by courtesy of Professor M Harboe, Rikshospitalet, Oslo.)

into the gel, a precipitin line forms, if the antisera recognises an antigenic site, giving rise to a number of well-defined peaks in proportion to the complexity of the original sample (Figure 9.7). The area under the peaks is proportional to the concentration of the antigen.

Salient Features of Immunoprecipitation in Gels

The quantitative precipitin test measures the total amount of reacting antibodies and antigen and is not useful for assaying mixtures. Although as a quantitative test it is now largely superseded, it has been a useful analytical tool for providing information about specificities of reactions and the nature of antigenic determinants. Unlike immunoprecipitation in solution, the immunoprecipitation in gels adds a spatial dimension allowing for specific identification of different components by position.

Because immunoprecipitation depends on multivalent complexes, it is really only suitable for the estimation of the larger molecules, like proteins. Sensitivity is such that these techniques can generally detect down to 1–5 µg of protein /ml. They have been used very successfully for the routine estimation of serum proteins like the immunoglobulins.

Diffusion techniques will take a longer time to reach a fully-defined immunoprecipitin line than the electrophoretic technique. The size of the molecule is also significant in that larger molecules will diffuse more slowly, thus extending the time. Mancini plates (single radial immunodiffusion) can take several days to complete, whereas rocket electrophoresis will take a few hours for a similar estimation.

The specificity of immunoprecipitation can be significantly reduced by non-specific lines arising from a number of factors. For example, haemolysed and lipaemic blood samples can give rise to spurious results and various bacterial polysaccharides can form non-antigen antibody precipitates.

The volume of antisera used is quite high with these techniques and monoclonal antibodies are often not suitable. A mixture of monoclonal antibodies can be used as a reagent in some cases.

Light Scattering Immunoassays

The concentration of formed immunocomplexes and thus, by inference, the concentration of either antigen or antibody can be measured using light scattering principles. Light falling on soluble molecules or particles in solution induce harmonic oscillation of their electrons in synchrony with the wavelength of the incident light. These oscillations then give rise to light emission at the same wavelength but the light is radiated in all directions. This phenomenon is known as light scattering, and the intensity of the scattered light is proportional to the concentration of particles.

Measurement of immunocomplexes using these principles is either by nephelometry or by turbidimetry.

Nephelometry

The technique of nephelometry involves the measurement of scattered light at an angle (often 90°) to the incident light (Figure 9.8). Material other than the specific antigen or antibody in the sample may give rise to 'background' scatter. Molecules such as proteins and lipids are common sources of interference and, in some cases, it may be necessary to remove interfering factors by some form of pretreatment

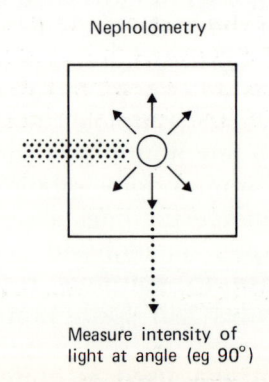

Figure 9.8 *Principle of nephelometry; the measurement of scattered light is directly proportional to the concentration of immune complexes formed from antibody and antigen.*

of the sample, e.g. centrifugation. More commonly, nephelometry is performed on samples as dilute as possible in order to minimise interference from the non-specific factors.

Nephelometry has a sensitivity similar to single radial immunodiffusion or electrophoretic immunoassay but analysis is achieved in a much shorter time. Table 9.2 compares times typical for the three techniques.

Table 9.2
Comparison of Times for Three Immunoprecipitation Methods

Single radial diffusion	1–3 days
Rocket immunoelectrophoresis	2–7 hours
Nephelometry	5–60 minutes

Nephelometry can be improved by measuring the scattered light at an angle forward of the 90° angle. The technique can also be automated, for example, with the use of centrifugal analysers and modern nephelometers often incorporate laser light sources. The instrumentation is expensive and so the technique will be most appropriate where there is a high throughput of samples.

Turbidimetry

Turbidimetry involves the measurement of transmitted light (Figure 9.9) in the same plane as the incident light and so is a measure of the reduction in light intensity due to the turbidity of the sample. The reduction in light intensity may

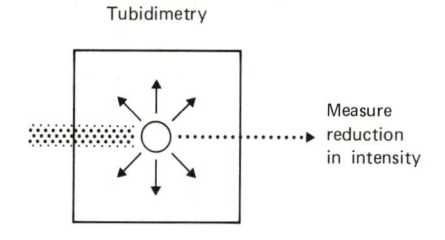

Figure 9.9 *Principle of turbidimetry; the measurement of transmitted light is indirectly proportional to the concentration of immune complexes.*

arise from absorption, reflection or scattering, and can be measured very simply in a spectrophotometer.

Turbidimetry, like nephelometry, is characterised by short reaction times but is more appropriate for higher concentrations of antigens having a sensitivity of approximately 0.5–1 µg/ml. The technique can be improved by the addition of polyethylene glycol (PEG 6000) at a concentration of 2–4% to give shorter reaction times and enhancement of the sensitivity. However, the addition of PEG may increase the sample background.

Turbidimetry can also be performed on automated centrifugal analysers where the use of kinetic measurements can reduce or eliminate problems arising from non-specific factors. Kinetic analysis is made by the difference in absorption between two timed measurements; for example, at 10 seconds and at 255 seconds.

Inhibition Nephelometry—Turbidimetry

Turbidimetry and nephelometry are generally limited to the measurement of large polyvalent antigens like the large immunoglobulins. However, techniques have been developed for measurement of small monovalent antigens. As haptens do not form immune complexes, techniques like nephelometry or turbidimetry are usually not suitable. But with modifications, small molecules can be measured by inhibition.

A polyvalent antigen is produced by covalently coupling several molecules of the monovalent antigen to a reasonably large protein like an albumin. An immune complex is produced when this synthesised polyvalent antigen is reacted with the relevant antibodies. This 'artificial' immune complex can be measured by nephelometry or turbidimetry. Concentrations of the small molecule or hapten will have an inhibitory effect on the formation of the immune complex and this will affect the nephelometric or turbidimetric measure (Figure 9.10). Using this approach it should prove possible to employ non-precipitating monoclonal antibodies as standard reagents.

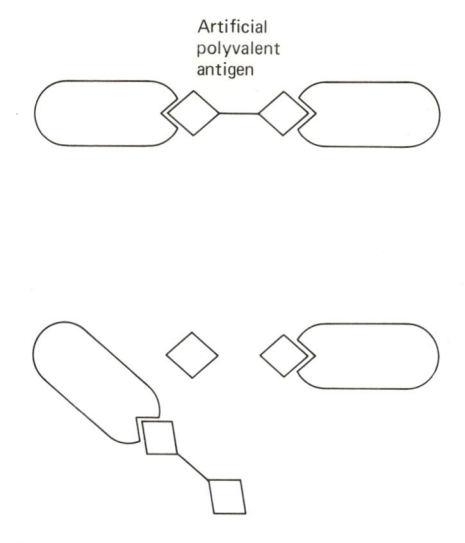

Figure 9.10 *Inhibition nephelometry or turbidimetry; the use of an artificial polyvalent antigen allows nephelometry or turbidimetry to be used to measure small molecules. Increasing concentrations of antigen inhibit the formation of immune complexes with the polyvalent antigen and consequently a change in signal.*

Latex Turbidimetry and Nephelometry

These techniques can also be extended by the judicious use of small particles, usually polystyrene and referred to as 'latex'. Antibodies or antigens coupled to the particles after reaction produce complexes that are detected with much greater efficiency. The use of particles for immunoassay detection is discussed in the next chapter.

Further Reading

Axelson N.H. ed. (1983). *Handbook of Immunoprecipitation-in-Gel Techniques*. Oxford: Blackwell Scientific Publications.

Price C.P., Spencer K., Whicher J. (1983). Light-scattering immunoassay of specific proteins: A review. *Ann. Clin. Biochem*; **20**:1–14.

CHAPTER TEN

Particle and Agglutination Immunoassays

Red Blood Cells

Red blood cells have been used as labels for monitoring and quantifying the immune reaction since the beginning of this century. They have been used extensively to elucidate the complement reaction and to quantify cell surface markers. Red blood cell labelled antigens and antibodies were the basis of the haemagglutination immunoassay techniques of Coombs (1945). Haemagglutination immunoassays had been one of the major types of immunoassay methods for a number of years, when Yalow and Berson published work leading to their development of radioimmunoassay. Although haemagglutination immunoassays lack the sensitivity of some of the immunoassays developed later, they have continued in use, a token of their practicality and usefulness.

Direct Haemagglutination Immunoassays

Red blood cells have certain endogenous antigenic binding sites which will react with specific antibodies. In the presence of these antibodies, red blood cells will agglutinate (Figure 10.1); haemagglutination being simply the agglutination of the red blood cells. The degree of agglutination is proportional to the amount of specific antibody present. The direct haemagglutination immunoassay has been the basis of much of the work on blood groups analysis.

Passive Haemagglutination (Indirect Haemagglutination)

Red blood cells can be pretreated so that they passively absorb exogenous antigens. This was done originally by

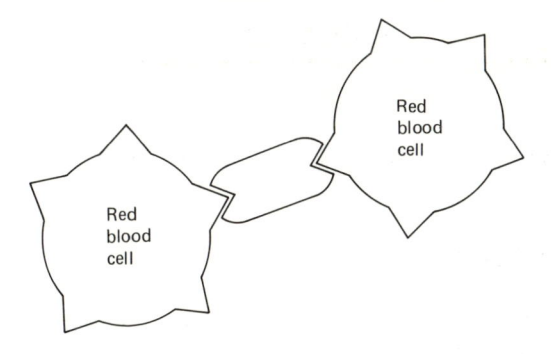

Figure 10.1 *Haemagglutination; specific antibodies to endogenous antigenic sites on red blood cells cause the cells to agglutinate. The degree of agglutination is a measure of the specific antibodies.*

Boyden (1951) with tannic acid giving the so-called tanned red cells. After absorption of antigen by the tanned red cell, haemagglutination of these cells is a measure of antibodies specific to the absorbed antigen (Figure 10.2). This most common type of haemagglutination immunoassay is referred to by the terms passive or indirect.

Because of troubles with leaching of antigen from the surface of tanned red cells and non-specific adsorption, various techniques have been developed to improve and optimise antigen coupling. Chromic chloride and glutaraldehyde covalent coupling techniques have been used successfully to give more satisfactory antigen-red blood cell products.

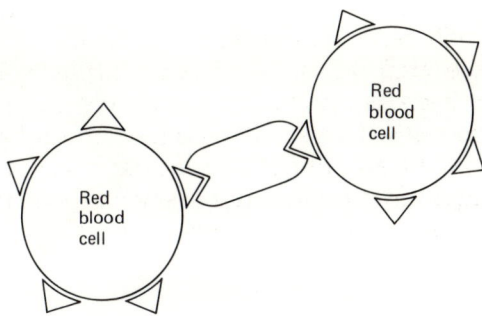

Figure 10.2 *Passive haemagglutination; exogenous antigens can be absorbed onto red blood cells. Agglutination of these cells is a measure of antibodies specific to the absorbed antigens.*

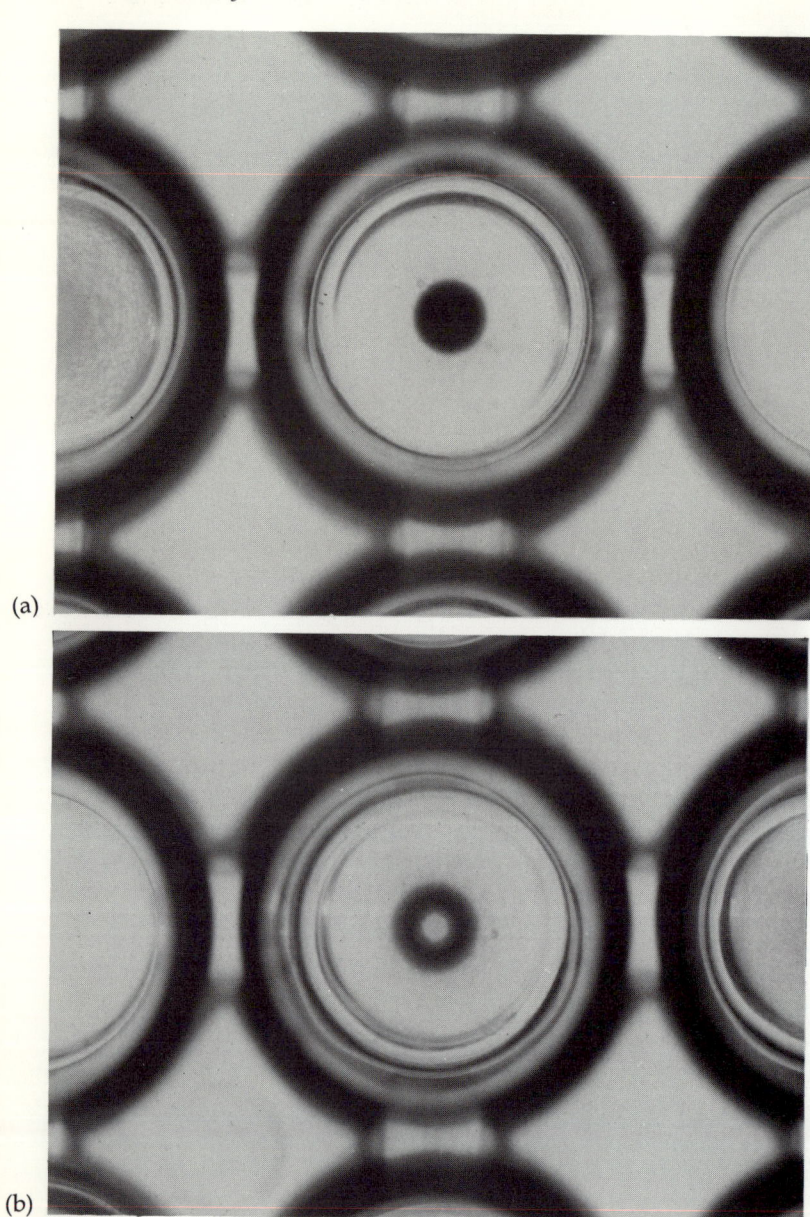

Figure 10.3 Degrees of haemagglutination; in this test (passive haemagglutination) for hepatitis B antigen, the stages are: (a) negative result, (b) very weak positive, (c) weak positive, (d) positive. (By courtesy of Ian Cayzer, Wellcome Diagnostics, Beckenham, UK.)

Particle and Agglutination Immunoassays 127

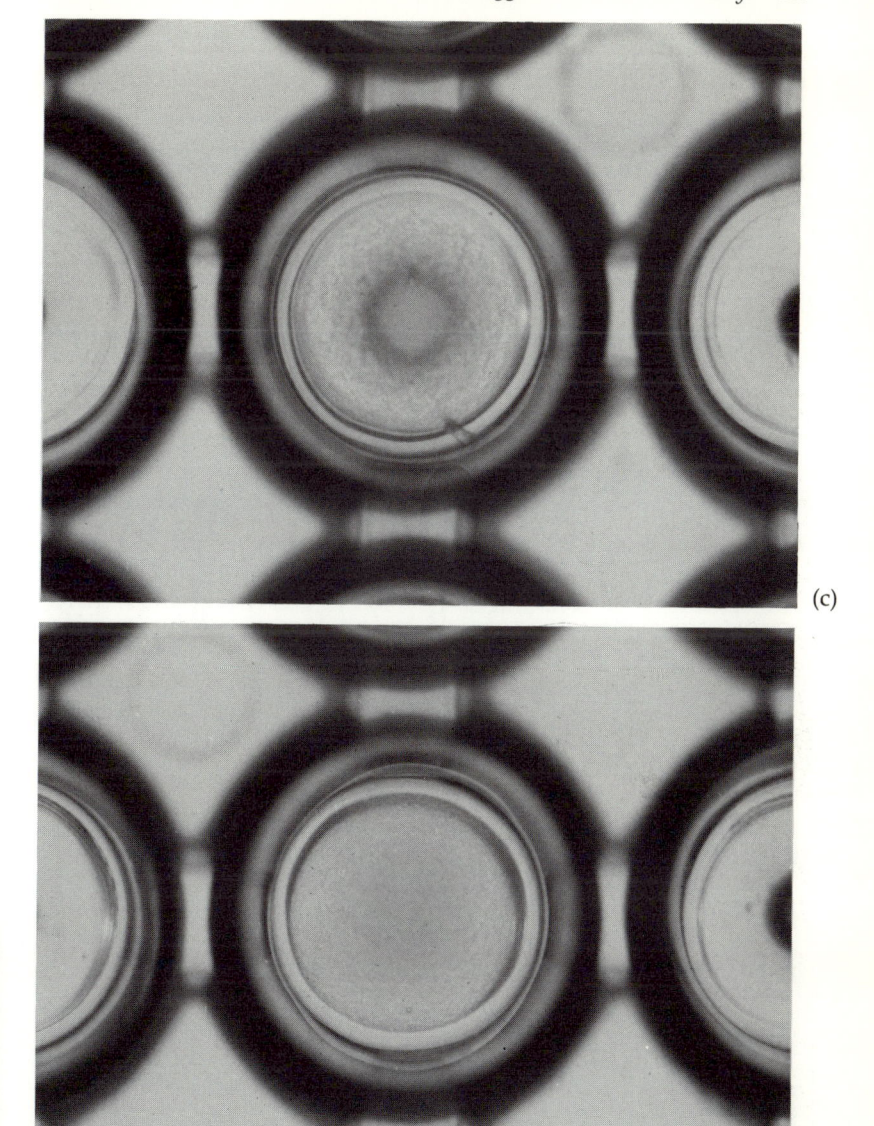

(c)

(d)

128 Immunoassay

Some antigens will bind strongly to untreated red blood cells; for example, many polysaccharide antigens from bacterial cell walls. For this reason, passive haemagglutination techniques have been used extensively to monitor antibodies to various bacterial infections and for various epidemiological studies.

Haemagglutination techniques can be used without any sophisticated instrumentation and the results are evaluated by eye. Examples of the various stages of haemagglutination are shown in Figure 10.3. The degree of haemagglutination is obviously subjective, although the difference between a positive result and a negative result is unequivocal. This qualitative assessment can be readily quantified by assaying samples at a series of dilutions (Figure 10.4). The highest dilution to give a positive result serves as a quantitative measure of potency.

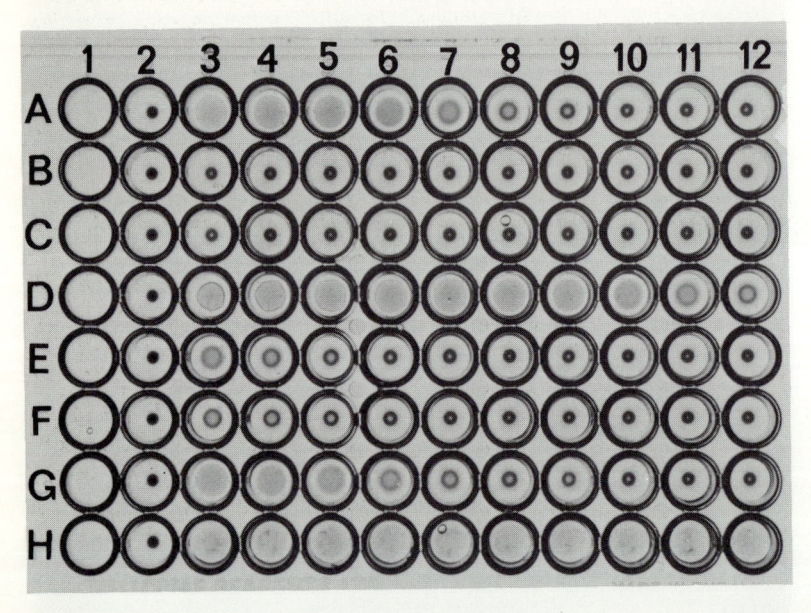

Figure 10.4 *Haemagglutination assay in microtitre wells; in this test for thyroglobulin autoantibodies, each row (vertically, A–H) represents a different serum sample at doubling dilutions from 1:10 column (3–12). Columns 1 and 2 are blanks and controls, respectively. Rows D and H show positive results for samples at a dilution >1:5120. Rows B and C show samples with negative results. (By courtesy of Ian Cayzer, Wellcome Diagnostics, Beckenham, UK.)*

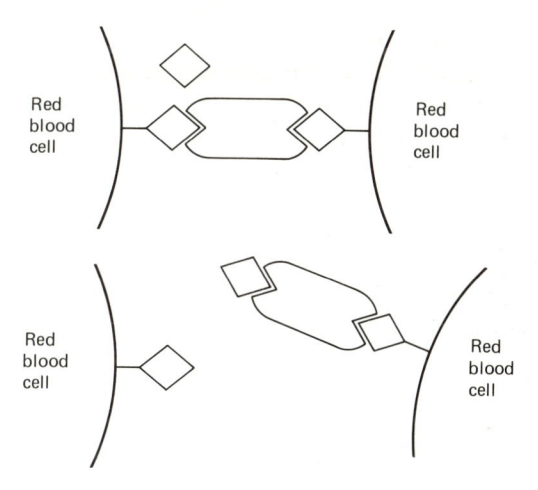

Figure 10.5 *Inhibition haemagglutination; haemagglutination (and passive haemagglutination) can be used to measure antigen. Increasing concentrations of antigen inhibits the agglutination of the cells in the presence of a fixed concentration of antibody.*

Haemagglutination Inhibition Immunoassays

In addition to these methods for the quantitation of antibodies, passive haemagglutination can be used to measure antigens (Figure 10.5). This method involves essentially an inhibition of haemagglutination. In the absence of antigen to be measured, the antibodies will bind only to the red cell conjugated antigen giving rise to maximum haemagglutination. The increasing concentration of antigen in the sample will react with an increasing proportion of antibodies, producing a decreasing proportion of haemagglutination. The samples may be reacted with antibody before the subsequent reaction of the excess antibody with red cell labelled antigen.

Reverse Passive Haemagglutination

The more common procedure for detecting and quantifying antigen by haemagglutination techniques is with the anti-

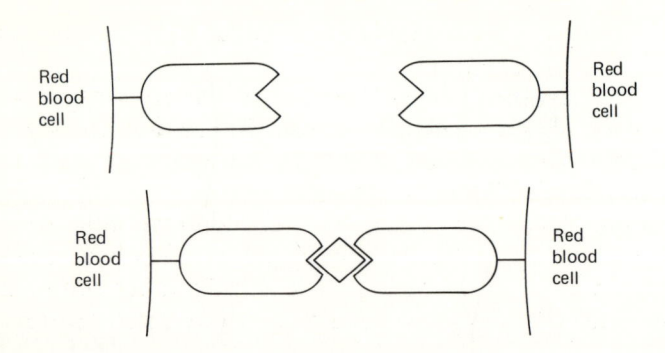

Figure 10.6 *Reverse passive haemagglutination; antigen is measured by the degree of agglutination of the antibody-red blood cell reagent. Increasing concentrations of antigen cause increasing degrees of agglutination.*

body absorbed or coupled to red blood cells. The red cell labelled antibodies are then agglutinised by antigen (Figure 10.6) and the procedure is referred to as reverse passive haemagglutination. Increasing concentrations of antigen will cause a proportional increase in the degree of haemagglutination.

Salient Features of Haemagglutination

Much of the early work on haemagglutination was carried out with sheep erythrocytes. The use of red blood cells from other species can improve the haemagglutination techniques. For example, the assay, illustrated in Figure 10.4, is based on turkey red blood cells which are nucleated and may have better properties for stability and more well-defined haemagglutination. The fragility of prepared red blood cells is a problem in that they may not store well. For example, most red blood cell labelled antibodies have a relatively short shelf life of 2–3 weeks. Developments are under way to improve the stability of red cell reagents and it does seem likely that the shelf life will be increased.

Perhaps one of the most useful aspects of haemagglutination techniques is the simplicity of the technique. This means that the method can be used without instrumentation, and especially expensive detection systems. Although the end-point is subjective, the method can be used in a quantitative way as shown in Figure 10.4.

Another problem with haemagglutination assays is the prevalence of non-specific reactions. These do vary with red blood cells from different species, and is one of the advantages of the turkey erythrocyte.

Another early problem with red cell reagents was the leaching away from the erythrocyte of the adsorbed antibody or antigen. The problem has been considerably reduced by milder and more efficient covalent coupling procedures.

Haemolysis Immunoassays

Serum complement components have two interesting aspects that have been used in developing immunoassay methods. In the first place, complement factors bind to some immunoglobulins when aggregated or when antibodies are combined with their specific antigens. Secondly, the binding of complement factors to an antibody in combination with antigen on the surface of a red blood cell can lead to lysis of the blood cell (Figure 10.7). The complement-induced haemolysis occurs when the appropriate antibody is directed against an endogenous antigen or when the antigen is

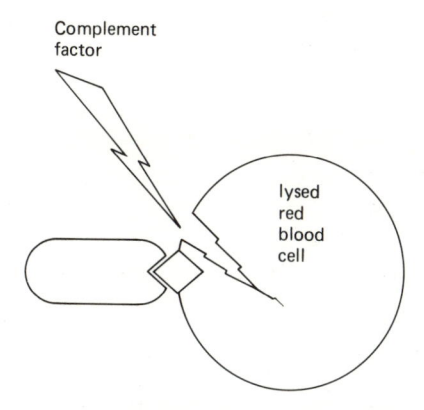

Figure 10.7 *Passive haemolysis assay; complement factors bind to antibody and antigen complexes. Where the antigen is on a blood cell, binding of complement causes lysis of the cell. The extent of haemolysis is a measure of antibody.*

adsorbed or coupled to the surface of the red cell. As with the terminology in haemagglutination techniques, these are referred to as direct haemolysis (endogenous antigen) and passive haemolysis (adsorbed or coupled antigen).

In the passive haemolysis immunoassay (Figure 10.7), the antibody to be detected or measured is reacted with a fixed amount of red cell–antigen reagent in the presence of an excess of serum complement. Thus, an increasing concentration of antibody will produce an increasing amount of haemolysis.

Passive Haemolysis Inhibition Assay (PHI)

Analagous to haemagglutination procedures, antigen can also be measured by the inhibition of passive haemolysis. Antigen in the sample will react with the antibody which will then bind complement, leaving proportionally less haemolysis of the red cell labelled antigen (Figure 10.8).

Complement Fixation Assays

In the conventional complement fixation assay, the reacted antibody and antigen bind complement factor with the complement present in excess. The residual unfixed comple-

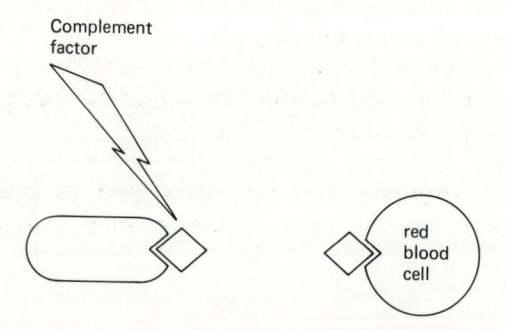

Figure 10.8 *Passive haemolysis inhibition assay; antigens can be measured in the haemolysis assay. Binding of antibodies by increasing concentrations of antigen binds complement factor, leading to less binding of complement factor to complexes with red blood cells, and subsequently less lysis.*

ment is then reacted with antibody-sensitised red blood cells. The greater the amount of residual complement, then the greater degree of haemolysis will result. The concentration of unreacted complement available to produce the haemolysis is inversely proportional to the concentration of reacted antibody and antigen. In this manner, complement fixation can provide the basis for quantitation of either antibody or antigen.

Salient Features of Haemolysis Immunoassay Methods

Haemolysis can be conveniently monitored using a simple spectrophotometer at 412 nm. As haemolysis proceeds, the red colour released from the lysed erythrocyte increases, and similarly, the absorption increases. It is also possible to monitor the lysis of red blood cells by the release of ^{51}Cr. The radioisotope of chromium must have been previously introduced into the erythrocyte.

Haemolysis can also be detected by the formation of haemolytic plaques from erythrocytes embedded in a gel. This procedure is usually carried out to detect cells such as specific lymphocyte cells which are secreting particular immunoglobulin antibodies. Both the cell population containing the particular cells and the erythrocytes are embedded in a gel. The secretion from each cell permeates the gel and any antibodies specific for the erythrocyte antigens in the presence of complement, also in the gel, give rise to haemolytic plaques, the so-called plaque-forming cell assay. This assay can be used to identify single antibody-secreting cells in large populations of other cells.

Analogous to other systems the relative positions of antigen and antibody can be interposed to give reverse passive haemolysis assays, reverse plaque-forming cell assays, etc.

Bacterial Plaque Assays

The haemolytic plaque-forming cell assay is a development of the bacterial plaque assay. This is an assay where bacteria were lysed following infection with specific viruses or bacteriophages. In this instance, the bacterial lysis gives rise to a plaque. This basic assay system has been used in a highly innovative way to monitor antibody–antigen reactions. Small antigens or haptens are covalently coupled to bacteriophage. This bacteriophage still retains the ability to infect bacterial cells. However, binding to the bacteriophage antigen by antibody restricts the bacteriophage and inhibits the infection and subsequent plaque formation. Reaction of the antibody with varying concentrations of sample antigen will give inversely proportional binding of antibody to the bacteriophage. This in turn gives a variable plaque formation and a consequent assay system. For those with the relevant skills this assay proved very sensitive, rivalling other very sensitive systems like radioimmunoassay.

Rosetting Reaction Assays

Rosetting reactions are essentially the agglutination of two different cell types; for example, red blood cells and lymphocytes. The assay can be directly applied for detection of antibodies to common antigenic sites on the two types of cell with formation of a rosette of, for example, the red cells agglutinated around the other cell type (for example, the lymphocyte). This type of assay has been used successfully to demonstrate the presence of blood cell type antigens on other cells. The two principal variants of the basic rosetting reaction assays are the direct antiglobulin rosette reaction (DARR), and the indirect antiglobulin rosette reaction (IARR). In these assays, the rosetting cell is coupled to either an antibody, i.e. direct or a second antibody, i.e. indirect (Figure 10.9).

Latex Particle Immunoassay

In an analogous way to the use of cells, latex particles can be used as labels for immunoassay reagents. Latex particles, made from polystyrene and about $0.8\,\mu m$ diameter, can be used to adsorb antibodies or antigens. Antigens adsorbed on

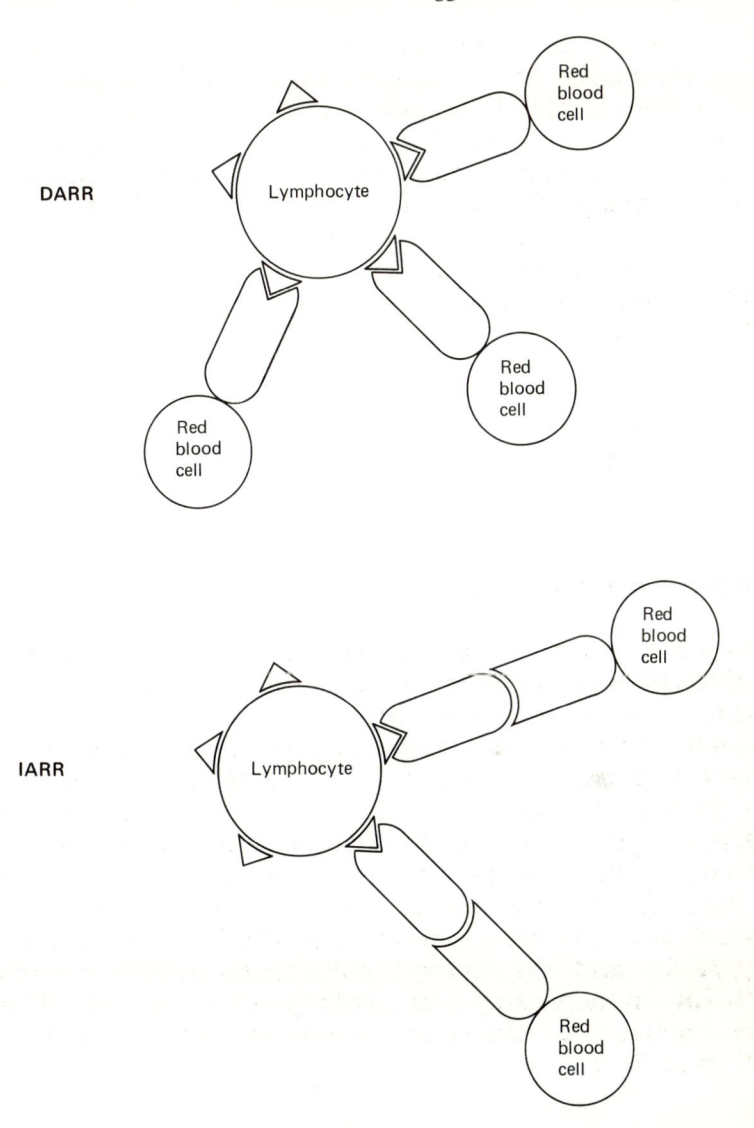

Figure 10.9 Rosetting reaction assays; formation of rosettes—agglutinations of two different cell types—can be used to measure antibodies for antigenic sites common to both cells. In the variations above (a) red blood cells coupled to specific antibodies are used to measure antigenic sites on the lymphocyte (direct antiglobulin rosetting reaction, DARR), (b) red blood cells coupled to anti-immunoglobulins are used to measure antibodies reacting with lymphocytes (indirect antiglobulin rosetting reaction, IARR).

136 *Immunoassay*

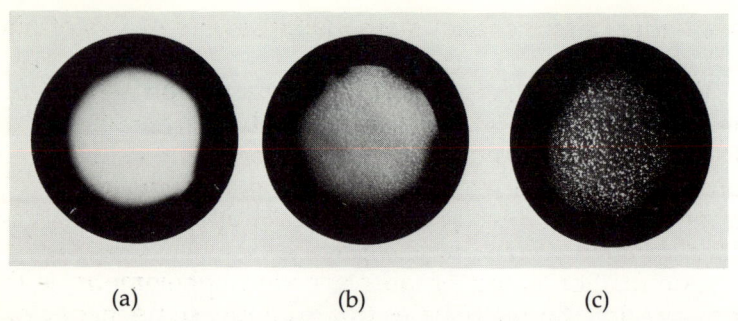

Figure 10.10 *Latex particle agglutination; in this test for rheumatoid factor the degrees of agglutination are: (a) negative result, (b) weak positive reaction, (c) strong positive reaction. (By courtesy of Ian Cayzer, Wellcome Diagnostics, Beckenham, UK.)*

to latex particles can be agglutinised by antibodies. Agglutination of latex particles gives distinctive patterns that can be read by eye (Figure 10.10). As with other qualitative and subjective detection systems, latex agglutination can be used to give quantitative or semiquantitative results by assaying samples at varying dilutions. Latex agglutination immunoassays, using antigen-coated particles, have been used to detect and determine various circulating autoimmune antibodies.

Antigen-coated particles reacting with a fixed concentration of antibody will give a latex agglutination inhibition immunoassay for antigens, and antibody-coated particles give a latex agglutination immunoassay directly proportional to the antigen concentration.

The most obvious advantages of latex particles over the use of red blood cells for agglutination is the stability of the reagents and a reduction in non-specific reactions.

Latex Particle Nephelometric and Turbidimetric Immunoassays

Latex particles coupled to antibodies or antigens have been used to refine nephelometric and turbidimetric immunoassay procedures (see p. 120, Chapter 9). The use of these latex particle reagents can improve the sensitivity of light scattering immunoassay methods by several orders of magnitude.

With the improvement in instrumentation over recent years (particularly the introduction of laser light sources and the reduction of the angle of measurement to a forward angle) latex particle nephelometry can reach sensitivities approximately 10 µg/litre compared to approximately 1 mg/litre for conventional nephelometry.

One further aspect of latex particle nephelometry is that non-precipitating antibodies (for example, some monoclonal antibodies) can be used as reagents.

As with the other agglutination assays, latex particle reagents can be used in an inhibition mode.

Particle Counting Immunoassays (PACIA)

Particle counting using small polystyrene latex particles with a defined size (usually 0·8 µm diameter), can be a precise detection system. Particle counters work on one of the basic methods, either measuring a change in electrical resistance, or a change in light transmission. The particles are streamed for counting and this means that they are useful as detection systems in continuous flow automated assay systems.

Particle counting has been applied successfully to the immunoassay of a number of antigens (PACIA). Reagents and samples are reacted together in a continuous flow system and the flow passes through a particle counter based on forward light scattering nephelometric measurements. The instrument is set to monitor particle sizes between 0·6 and 1·2 µm diameter only. Thus, interference from small particles, i.e. <0·6 µm, such as dust, chylomicra and lipoproteins, are minimised. Agglutinated particles are ignored as they would be >1·2 µm, i.e. at least 2 × 0·8 µm, and so, in theory, only unreacted particles are counted. This gives a measurement which is inversely proportional to the concentration of test substance.

The method does reduce the effects of non-specific interference and is capable of achieving a reasonable sensitivity on a par with RIA. It is also very suitable for automated immunoassays, although the instrumentation is costly.

Further Reading

Borsos T. (1981). Quantification of complement fixation by the C1 fixation and C1 fixation and transfer tests. In: *Methods in Enzymology, Vol. 74: Immunochemical Techniques, Part C.* Ch. 10, pp. 165–76. London: Academic Press.

Borsos T., Langone J.J. (1981). Detection of antigens and haptens by inhibition of passive immune hemolysis. In: *Methods in Enzymology, Vol. 74: Immunochemical Techniques, Part C*; Ch. 9, pp. 161–5. London: Academic Press.

Coombs R.R.A. (1981). Assays utilizing red cells as markers. In: *Immunoassays for the 80s.* (Voller A., Barlett A. Bidwell D., eds.) Ch. 3, pp. 17–34. Lancaster: MTP Press.

Lefkovits I., Pernis B. eds. (1979). *Immunological Methods.* London: Academic Press.

Masson P.L., Collet-Cassart D., Magnusson C.G., Sindic C.J.M., Cambiaso C.L. (1981). Particle counting immunoassay (PACIA): An automated non-radioisotopic immunoassay method, suitable for antigens, haptens, antibodies and immune complexes. In: *Immunoassays for the 80s.* (Voller A., Bartlett A., Bidwell D., eds.) Ch. 4, pp. 35–41. Lancaster: MTP Press.

Masson P.L., Cambiaso C.L., Collet-Cassart D., Magnusson C.G.M., Richards C.B., Sindic C.J.M. (1981). Particle counting immunoassay (PACIA). In: *Methods in Enzymology, Vol. 74: Immunochemical Techniques, Part C.* Ch. 6, pp. 106–39. London: Academic Press.

Thompson R.A. ed. (1981). *Techniques in Clinical Immunology.* Oxford: Blackwell Scientific Publications.

CHAPTER ELEVEN

Comparison, Application and Enhancement

Introduction

An impression is often given that a choice between different types of immunoassay procedures can be made on the basis of personal taste and preference. This would rarely be the case. Invariably, there is a range of factors that need to be considered for each particular application. Consideration of these factors often prejudices the choice to such an extent that only one, or possibly two, of the methods are really appropriate. It then becomes more apparent that methods have been developed for specific applications and not as alternative procedures to be followed on the basis of arbitrary predeliction.

The factors that have a bearing on the choice of immunoassay procedure include: concentration of analyte; range of concentrations; chemical nature of analyte; type of sample; type of test (quantitative or semi-quantitative); availability and quality of reagents; cost and technical complexity.

Concentration of Analyte

One of the first factors to be evaluated is that of concentration. For any given analyte it will be necessary to decide what target concentration, or range of concentrations, is required. Each type of immunoassay procedure will only cover a limited concentration range, being unsuitable for measurements above or below this specified range.

An approximate guide to the comparative range of concentrations for different immunoassay methods is given in Figure 11.1. This guide classifies methods according to the particular type of label used. The range and sensitivity of any immunoassay method depends on not only the type of label

140 *Immunoassay*

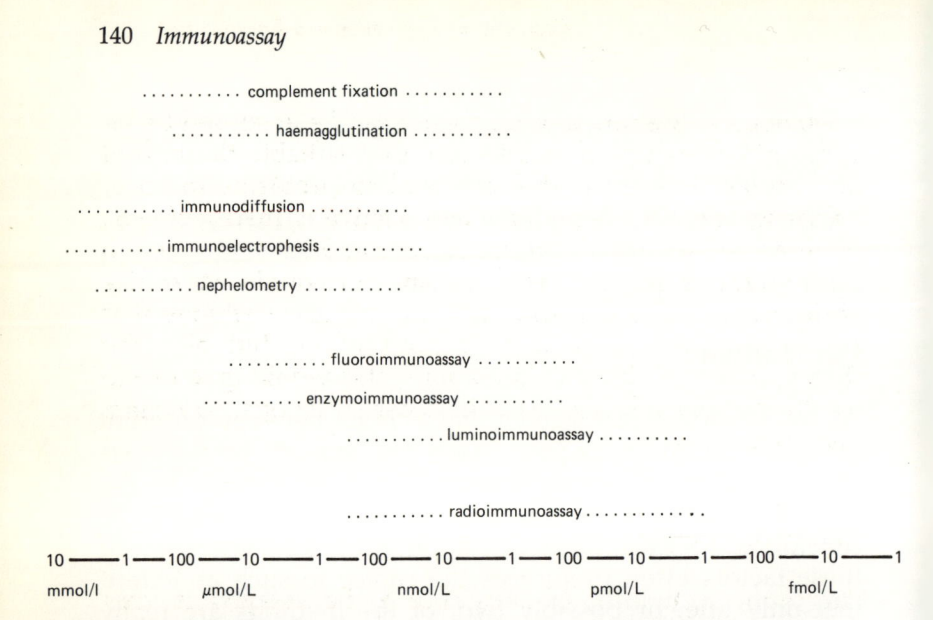

```
........... complement fixation ...........
      ........... haemagglutination ...........

........... immunodiffusion ...........
........... immunoelectrophesis ...........
........... nephelometry ...........

         ........... fluoroimmunoassay ...........
         ........... enzymoimmunoassay ...........
                ........... luminoimmunoassay ..........

              ........... radioimmunoassay ............
```

10——1——100——10——1——100——10——1——100——10——1——100——10——1
mmol/l   μmol/L   nmol/L   pmol/L   fmol/L

Figure 11.1 *Comparison of the concentration ranges of different immunoassays; these ranges are only an approximate guide.*

used, but also on many other factors. So this comparison is only valid in a very broad sense.

In general, the heterogeneous assays (those with a separation step) have greater sensitivity than the homogeneous assays (those with no separation step). Thus, the homogeneous assays should only be considered for application at higher concentrations.

Range of Assay

The range of concentrations over which measurement is required is another aspect which influences the decision on which type of assay system to use. The excess reagent methods, or immunometric assays, have a greater working range for a given sample volume than the limited reagent methods, i.e. immunoassays. The greater working range of the immunometric assays is usefully illustrated by its precision profile, compared with that for the equivalent immunoassay (see Figure 4.8). Of course, the biphasic response seen in some assays may severely limit the useful range.

Obviously, the range of any assay can be extended by an appropriate change in sample size or a suitable dilution of the sample. However, this can lead to problems in some circumstances. The assay may be sensitive to matrix effects, such as those arising from large variations in protein concentrations. In such cases, a change in sample size or use of different dilutions could give rise to measurements that not only reflect the analyte concentrations but also the change in matrix. In some situations, this would give rise to results that are too high and, in other situations, to results that are too low.

Nature of Analyte

The type, or nature, of substance to be assayed is very significant in choosing the most appropriate method. Most analytes can be broadly categorised on the basis of size, outlined in Table 11.1.

Table 11.1
Size of Analyte

Small molecules	Molecular weight <5000
Medium molecules	Molecular weight >5000–50 000
Large molecules	Molecular weight >50 000–2 × 10^6
Particles	Membrane fragments; immune complexes
Cells	Bacteria; tissue cells; viruses

Molecules with low molecular weights are usually measured by some form of immunoassay or an inhibition type of immunometric assay. As the prospective analytes increase in molecular size, other methods become suitable. Assays that depend on immunoprecipitin, for example, generally require analytes with molecular size above 20–30 000 for easy operation.

Very large molecules are easily measured by immunoprecipitation methods and light scattering techniques, like nephelometry. Particles or cells can only be assayed by those methods that do not depend on the solubility of the analyte. A general guide to the application of the different techniques is given in Table 11.2.

Table 11.2
Guide to Application of Different Techniques—Based on Size of Analyte

	Small	Medium	Large	Particle	Cell
Immunoassay	√	√	√		
Immunometric		√	√		
Immunometric (inhibition)	√				
Agglutination		√	√	√	√
Immunodiffusion		√	√	√	
Complement fixation		√	√	√	
ELISA or RAST type of immunometric				√	√
Light Scattering		√	√	√	

Heterogeneity of the antigen is a particular problem that causes difficulties in the interpretation of many methods. Where the antigen population exhibits marked heterogeneity, such as fragment and complex formation, resolution is often possible using techniques that rely on a dual characterisation of the antigen. A useful example is the immunoelectrophoretic technique. The antigen is analysed on the basis of both its electrophoretic migration and its immunological reactivity. The crossed immunoelectrophoretic technique (described on p. 117, Chapter 9) is particularly useful for the quantitation of very heterogeneous antigen populations. It can also be used to study dissociation and association phenomena, which are, as it were, variants of heterogeneity.

Obviously, immunoelectrophoresis is not practical for antigens that do not migrate in the electrophoretic field; other methods, like double immunodiffusion, are more appropriate.

Another particularly interesting aspect relating to the nature of analytes is toxicity. Where the antigen is toxic, care must be exercised with its handling. An interesting example is provided by the measurement of a clostridium botulinum toxin. These extremely toxic substances are best assayed using techniques requiring minimal concentrations of antigen. The concentrations of antigen used during labelling procedures would necessarily preclude the use of labelled antigen methods for this particular application. Consequently, the labelled antibody methods, particularly the most sensitive ones, reduce or eliminate the hazards of handling high concentrations of toxic material.

Type of Sample

The type of sample in which the analyte is to be measured can have some bearing on the method used. The nature of the sample can vary from the very complex, as in biological fluids like serum, urine or saliva, to the relatively simple, as in solvent extracts or aqueous washings. Although all the immunoassay methods can be used to analyse complex samples, there are some pertinent points to be made that limit use in particular circumstances.

Techniques that depend on measurement of light, such as nephelometry, turbidimetry or fluorimetry, will be prone to error if samples are turbid or opaque. This can arise from a number of causes, but common examples are lipaemia and haemolysis in samples of blood. The degree to which this is a problem depends to some extent on whether the light is measured in a restricted direction, as in nephelometry, or whether the total light emitted is measured, as in some luminometers. The problem is relatively insignificant where light is detected from all around the sample, but will be much more significant for directional detection.

The suitability of different labels depends to a considerable extent on the relevant background measurements in samples. Radioisotopic labels are very suitable for measurements in many complex samples because of the extremely low (or absence of) background radioactivity. However, complex fluids, like serum or urine, may have high backgrounds with respect to certain measurements, like fluorescence. The need to increase the analytical signal, in relation to the background signal, will necessarily restrict the use of these susceptible techniques to the measurement of higher concentrations. Although, for simple samples with low backgrounds, the technique may show greater sensitivity.

Mention of numerous other factors in samples, like pH and ionic strength, that affect specific labels, can be found in the relevant chapters.

Requirements of the Test

Two general parameters of tests are the degree of quantitation required and the time necessary for completion of the analyses. Sometimes these two parameters are related in an inverse way. For example, a qualitative or semi-quantitative result may be obtained quickly, whilst a quantitative result can take much longer.

Where it is only necessary to demonstrate the presence or absence of a particular analyte, a qualitative assay will suffice. Most of the techniques available can be used in a qualitative or semi-quantitative mode. However, where no exacting degree of quantitation is required, attention should be given to those assay systems that require little or no instrumentation, such as the visual colour reaction with enzyme labels or simple immunodiffusion techniques.

These systems invariably require the least capital investment to implement. It should be mentioned that some techniques necessarily lend themselves to precise quantitation, such as the radiolabelled immunoassays or immunometric assays.

The question of time or length of assay must be governed to some extent by other requirements, such as necessary precision and accuracy. In general, the limited reagent assays (the immunoassays) will require a longer time to complete than excess reagent assays (the immunometric assays). An immunoassay may require an overnight reaction time, whilst the immunometric assay, for the same substance, may only take a few hours.

The different types of immunoprecipitation methods are particularly time dependent. For example, where single radial immunodiffusion may take three days for some of the larger molecules, the rocket technique can produce results in a few hours, and nephelometry in a much shorter time, from five minutes to one hour.

Availability and Quality of Reagents

A good supply of purified antigen is necessary for all of the labelled antigen immunoassay methods. This is one of the reasons why they are most frequently used to assay the lower molecular weight substances. These antigens are often readily synthesised, and thus are available in large amounts and with a good standard of purity. The purified labelled antigen can confer good specificity to an assay, even when used in conjunction with a heterogeneous population of antibodies.

The labelled antibody methods can be used where the antigen is in scarce supply. Relatively impure antigens can be used as the immunosorbent reagent in RAST, where crude allergens can be used, and ELISA, where crude antigens can be absorbed to the polystyrene surface.

In general, the amount of antisera used in immunoassays varies to some extent with the application and affinity of antibody involved in the reaction. Where low concentrations of analyte are being measured and the antibodies have a high avidity, i.e. where the equilibrium constant is high, the volume of antisera used is, for the most part, small; a few microlitres being sufficient for many thousands of anlayses. Conversely, a larger volume of antisera is used where high concentrations are measured and the avidity is low. Because the immunometric assays require the antibodies to be purified for labelling, they invariably require greater amounts of antisera than the corresponding immunoassays.

The non-labelled immunoassay methods usually have a requirement for large amounts of monospecific antisera. The degree of monospecificity is greater for techniques like nephelometry, where characterisation is solely a function of the immunological reagent, than it is for immunodiffusion, and even less so for immunoelectrophoretic techniques, where characterisation involves additional factors.

The quantity of reagent used in any assay is often related to the reaction time. It is an inverse relationship, with fast assays usually using more material than slow ones. For example, nephelometry may require about five times the quantity of antisera used for analogous immunodiffusion methods. Nephelometry also requires antisera with higher avidity than those used in immunoelectrophoretic or immunodiffusion techniques.

Cost and Technical Complexity

Technical complexity is very relative in the sense that where certain skills exist, the relevant techniques are considered simple, and where these skills are absent the same techniques will be considered very difficult. On this basis, it is reasonable to find some techniques more generally associated with certain disciplines. For example, it is not uncommon to find radioisotopes used more frequently in the disciplines of physics and nuclear medicine, whilst immunoprecipitation methods are more common in immunology. Undoubtedly, the appeal of different techniques can be related to an understanding of the principles involved and the technical skills practised. Notwithstanding, some immunoassay methods undoubtedly are less technically complex than others.

The technical skills involved in any method can be divided into three areas: reagent preparation, analytical procedure and, finally, measurement. Many specific immunological reagents are readily available from a number of commercial suppliers. Reagent preparation invariably requires considerable experience and often involves technically complex steps. Where possible, it is better to purchase the characterised and purified reagents from reputable suppliers. The preparation of radioisotopic labels is a particular example that requires special attention. It is usually necessary, in these instances, to use specially equipped laboratories for preparation and purification of the label. Obviously, the additional expense that would be involved in this makes the purchase of prepared reagents more attractive for many laboratories. The characterisation of reagents, an essential part of their preparation, is usually best left to the experienced laboratory or, at least, based on the findings of these laboratories.

The analytical procedures for many of the methods are relatively simple, which, of course, is one of the main advantages of immunoassay methods. However, a few techniques require more skill than the simple pipetting steps usually involved in immunoassay practice; for example, the pouring and casting of gels for immunoprecipitation.

It is in the measurement that the different degrees of technical complexity in various methods becomes marked. For some of the procedures, only an appraisal by eye is required, as with latex agglutination, haemagglutination and some enzyme colour reactions. For other assays, simple instrumentation, such as a basic spectrophotometer, colorimeter or gamma-counter is used; whilst for some methods, more sophisticated instrumentation, like a polarisation fluorimeter, is introduced. An indication of the different degrees of instrumentation involved in various immunoassay methods is given in Table 11.3.

Table 11.3

Type of immunoassay method	Degree of instrumentation
Latex agglutination	None necessary
Haemagglutination	
Immunodiffusion	
ELISA (semi-quantitative)	
Immunoelectrophoretic methods	Electrophoresis
Turbidimetry	Spectrophotometer (simple)
Enzyme-labelled assays	
—homogeneous	Colorimeter
—heterogeneous	Colorimeter and centrifuge*
Radiolabelled assays	Counter and centrifuge* (simple and unrefrigerated)
Nephelometry	Nephelometer
Fluoroimmunoassays	Fluorimeter
	Fluorimeter and centrifuge*
	Polarisation fluorimeter
	Fluorimeter with time-resolved measurements
Luminescent immunoassays	Luminometer and centrifuge*
Automation with high throughput of samples	Additional instrumentation for automated reagent addition, separation and detection

*Alternatively, other method of separation, e.g. magnets or filtration.

The cost of running immunoassay methods is mainly related to the use of instrumentation and its degree of sophistication. Reagents, even when purchased directly, need cost only a few pence per test. Of course, this cost does escalate where the volume of reagents used is very high, as in nephelometry. The capital cost of instruments can vary from a few hundred pounds for a simple gamma-counter or a colorimeter to many thousands, primarily depending on the degree of automation involved or the degree of sensitivity required.

Applications

A brief summary from the variety of applications of immunoassay methods, together with commonly used methods for each application, is given in Table 11.4. This summary illustrates well the potential advantages of immunoassay methods. It also serves to assist in choosing a particular method for a specific application.

Table 11.4

Type of immunoassay method	Examples of application
Latex agglutination	Early diagnosis of pregnancy—detection of human chorionic gonadotrophin (HCG) in urine (e.g. human and mares)
	Detection of rheumatoid factor (auto-antibodies to human IgG) in blood
	Presence of antibodies to thyroglobulins in serum from subjects with auto-immune thyroiditis
	C reactive protein detection and semi-quantitation in human serum
	Streptococcal grouping by specific antigens
	Fibrinogen degradation products in serum or urine
Haemolysis	Antibodies to rubella in serum
Complement fixation	Identification of viral infections by detection of antibodies, e.g. influenza A and B, measles, *Mycoplasma pneumoniae* and rubella
Haemagglutination	Detection of auto-antibodies to thyroglobulin and thyroid microsomal antigens to diagnose auto-immune thyroiditis
	Diagnosis of toxoplasmosis—antibodies to *Toxoplasma gondii*
	Identification of viral infections,

Table 11.4 (*continued*)

Type of immunoassay method	Examples of application
	e.g. measuring antibodies to measles, rubella (humans) and rinderpest
	Viral infections in infected fowl, e.g. detection of *Mycoplasma gallisepticum*, *Mycoplasma synoviae*
	Hepatitis B—detection in blood of hepatitis B antigen
Rosetting	Detection of complement (C_4) receptors on lymphocyte surface membranes (rosetted with red blood cells)
	Tissue typing
	Surface virus antigens on infected cells
Turbidimetry	Measurement of specific serum proteins, e.g. albumin, transferrin, IgA, IgG, IgM, α-acid glycoprotein, haptoglobulin, C reactive protein (CRP)
Nephelometry	Measurement of specific serum proteins
	Immunoglobulins
	Rheumatoid factor
Immunoelectrophoresis	Immunoglobulin components in serum, e.g. myeloma proteins and in macroglobulinaemia
	Reactive immunoglobulins against foot and mouth
Crossed immunoelectrophoresis	Heterogeneity in immunoglobulins
	Diagnosis of systemic candidosis, pneumococcal infections, meningococcal infections
Electroimmunoassay (rockets)	Quantitation of specific serum proteins, e.g. albumin, thyroid-binding globulin, IgA, IgG, IgM,

Table 11.4 (*continued*)

Type of immunoassay method	Examples of application
	pre-albumin, orosomucoid, cerulaplasmin, α_1-antitrypsin, α_2-macroglobulin, haptoglobulin, transferrin, C_3 complement
Single radial immunodiffusion	Quantitation of immunoglobulins
Double immunodiffusion	Quantitation of immunoglobulins
	Detection of antibodies in infections, e.g. swine vesicular diseases, rinderpest, canine viral hepatitis, distemper, 'blue-tongue' virus
	Specificity of antibodies
	Measurement of antinuclear antibodies
Luminescent immunoassays	Measurement of steroids in plasma, e.g. progesterone, oestradiol-17β and testosterone
	Measurement of steroid conjugates in urine, e.g. oestrone and oestriol glucuronides, pregnanediol glucuronide
	Measurement of thyroid-stimulating hormone (TSH) in serum
Fluoroimmunoassays —Homogeneous	Monitoring of therapeutic drugs, e.g. carbamazepine, phenytoin, gentamycin
	Measurement of hormones, e.g. cortisol, human placental lactogen (HPL), human chorionic gonadotrophin (HCG)
	Albumin in urine, serum and cerebrospinal fluid (CSF)
	Measurement of proteins, e.g. immunoglobulins, C reactive protein
—Heterogeneous	Measurement of therapeutic drugs,

Table 11.4 (continued)

Type of immunoassay method	Examples of application
	e.g. gentamycin, tobramycin, procainamide, N-acetyl procainamide, propanolol
	Measurement of steroid hormones, e.g. cortisol, 17α OH progesterone, pregnancy oestriol
	Measurement of immunoglobulins, human placental lactogen (HPL)
	Measurement of alphafoetoprotein (AFP) in amniotic fluid
Immunofluorometric —Time resolved	Measurement of human chorionic gonadotrophin (HCG), thyroid stimulating hormone (TSH), alphafoetoprotein (AFP) and ferritin
—Homogeneous	Immunoglobulins
Enzymeimmunoassay —Homogeneous	Monitoring of therapeutic drugs, e.g. amphetamine, N-acetyl procainamide, carbamazepine, diazepam, digoxin, gentamicin, lidocaine, methotrexate, morphine, phenytoin, phenobarbital, propanolol, tobramycin, theophylline
—Heterogeneous	Measurement of proteins, e.g. alphafoetoprotein (AFP)
Immunoenzymometric—ELISA	Detection of serological antibodies to infectious diseases, e.g. bacterial diseases (salmonella, vibriocholera, brucella abortus); mycotic diseases (aspergillus); viral diseases (rubella); parasitic diseases (malaria, schistosomiasis) used both for identification of infection and epidemiological studies
	Detection of infectious antigens, e.g. candida albicans, vibriocholera, hepatitis B

Table 11.4 (*continued*)

Type of immunoassay method	Examples of application
	Detection of both antigens and antibodies in infectious disease in animals, e.g. foot and mouth virus, African swine fever
	Detection of plant viruses, e.g. citrus tristeza, plum pox, lettuce mosaic, tobacco ringspot, soybean mosaic, potato leaf roll
	Detection of infectious organisms in food, e.g. staphylococcal enterotoxin
	Measurement of oncofoetal proteins, e.g. alphafoetoprotein (AFP), carcinoembryonic antigen (CEA)
Radioimmunoassay	Measurement of hormones in most biological fluids (viz. serum, plasma, urine, saliva, cerebrospinal fluid) e.g. insulin, thyroid hormones (T4 and T3), steroids, pituitary hormones (prolactin, growth hormone, luteinising hormone (LH), follicle stimulating hormone (FSH), thyroid stimulating hormone (TSH)
	Measurement of vitamins, e.g. B_{12}, folate
	Measurement of drugs, e.g. digoxin, acetylcholine, metyrapone, haloperidol, morphine
	Measurement of specific enzymes and iso-enzymes, e.g. creatine kinases, pancreatic amylase, muscle pyruvate kinase
	Measurement of serum proteins, e.g. ferritin, alphafoetoprotein (AFP), blood clotting proteins (β thromboglobulin, platelet factor 4), myoglobulin

Table 11.4 (continued)

Type of immunoassay method	Examples of application
Immunoradiometric assay	Specific and sensitive measurement of protein hormones, e.g. thyroid stimulating hormone (TSH), luteinising hormone (LH), follicle stimulating hormone (FSH), prolactin, growth hormone
	Specific measurement using two discrete antibodies reacting with two distinct sites on hormone molecule, e.g. IRMA for parathyroid hormone (PTH) and adrenocorticotrophic hormone (ACTH) dependent on both N and C terminals of peptides
	Quantitation of oncofoetal proteins, e.g. alphafoetoprotein (AFP), carcinoembryonic antigen (CEA), human chorionic gonadotrophin (HCG)
	Quantitation of specific classes of antibodies (antibody class capture assay) for IgG, IgA and IgM
	Specific IgE assays for allergens (RAST) e.g. house dust mite and grass pollen, and relevant antibodies in affected subjects
	Measurement of proteins, e.g. ferritin, factor VIII, anti-haemophilic factor and Von Willebrand factor.
	Detection of serological antibodies to infectious diseases in humans and animals (see application in ELISA)

Enhancement

On occasions, it becomes necessary to amend or enhance existing methodology in order to improve the performance in some way or other. Quite often, increased specificity or

154 *Immunoassay*

sensitivity is required. In a basic text on immunoassay methods it is not possible to comment on all the current techniques for enhancing performance. However, it is useful to indicate some general areas with the use of a few selected examples.

The most obvious step to be taken in improving assays is through the use of purified antibodies or the selection of monoclonal antibodies. This has already been discussed to some extent in Chapter 5.

Where lack of specificity in the assay system is related to non-specific reactions of the whole antibody molecule, improvements can be achieved by the judicious use of Fab or F(ab)$_2$ fragments derived from the antibody.

Second antibodies used in separation steps and in indirect label methods often have poor specificity. Consequently, improvements in this area can be very fruitful in terms of enhanced performance. An example of the improvement in specificity following affinity chromatography of second antibody is detailed in Figure 11.2. Recent reports indicate that second antibodies raised to Fc or Fab fragments of immuno-

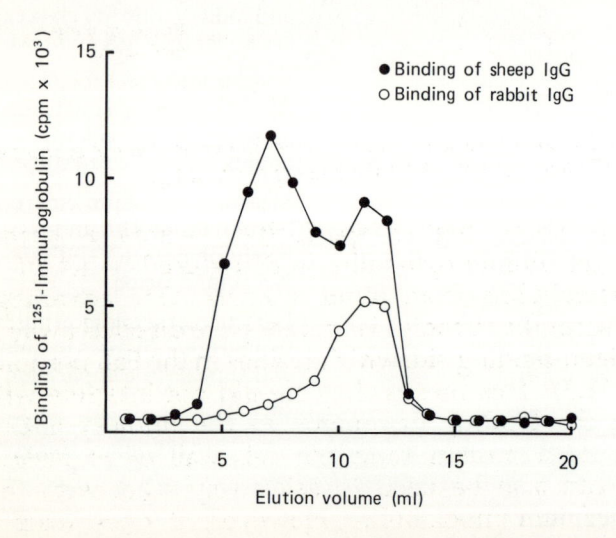

Figure 11.2 *Purification of antisheep second antibody by affinity chromatography; the elution profile indicates two populations of antibodies, one specific for sheep immunoglobulins and the other non-specific, as it reacts with both sheep and rabbit immunoglobulins.*

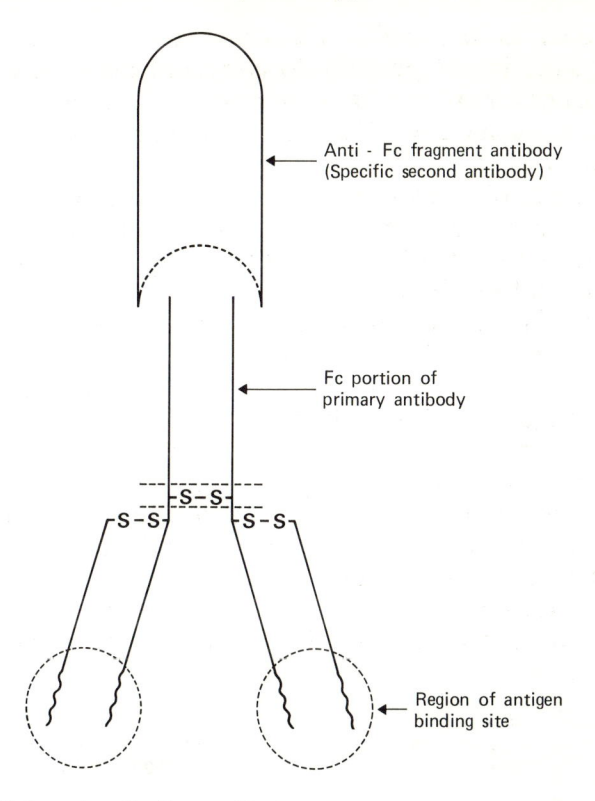

Figure 11.3 *Second antibodies specific for Fc fragments; the use of these specific second antibodies does not inhibit the binding of the antigen.*

globulins show higher specificity towards a particular species of immunoglobulin and reduced reaction with immunoglobulins from other animals. One advantage of anti-Fc second antibodies is that they are directed away from the antigen-binding site which resides in the Fab portion (see Figure 11.3). This means they should not interfere with or impede the binding of antigen to the primary antibody. Protein A, a protein from the cell wall of *Staphylococcus aureus*, can also be used to selectively react with the Fc region of immunoglobulin. However, it does react to a varying degree with immunoglobulins from many different species.

Enhancement of sensitivity can be achieved by amplification factors, such as increasing the number of labelled

156 Immunoassay

molecules bound to the reagent or by combining various techniques; for example, the use of radioactive substrates in enzyme-labelled assays.

Simply increasing the specific activity, i.e. the number of label groups per reagent molecule, frequently leads to loss of antigen-binding activity when the substitution reaches a certain level. An alternative approach is to use additional layers of reagents (as illustrated in Figure 11.4) each carrying more label. A cautionary note should be added here as this method may lead to increased non-specific measurements, and thus remove the advantage accrued from the increased signal.

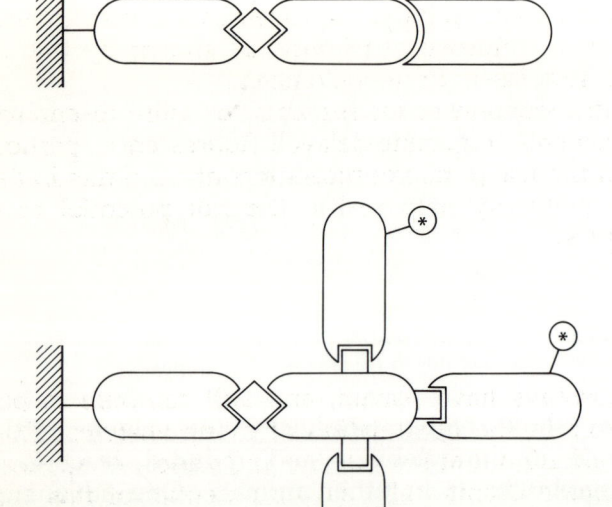

Figure 11.4 *Enhancement by label amplification; in these examples, the signal is increased by additional layers of labels (*). (Top) The signal with a labelled antibody is increased by the binding of a labelled anti-immunoglobulin. (Bottom) The antibody is modified by the conjugation of haptens. Labelled anti-hapten antibodies reacting with the haptens conjugated to the primary antibody increase the number of labels and hence the signal sometimes referred to as 'hapten sandwich labelling'. Biotin and avidin (the high affinity binding protein for biotin) can be substituted for hapten and anti-hapten antibody components, respectively.*

The use of radioactive labels in immunoelectrophoretic assays, like Laurell rockets, and subsequent autoradiography, can lead to a 25- to 50-fold improvement in sensitivity. A similar improvement can be found with enzyme- or fluorescent-labelled reagents. The use of radioisotopic substrates for enzyme-labelled reagents can also improve sensitivity many times, as indicated by the acronym USERIA (ultrasensitive enzymic radioimmunoassay). Essentially, an enzyme, e.g. alkaline phosphatase, is used with a radioactive substrate, e.g. ^{3}H-AMP, and the release of radioactive product, e.g. ^{3}H-adenosine, is measured following separation from excess substrate. Sensitivities are said to be improved by a factor of 1000. Fluorescent substrates can also be used in conjunction with enzyme-labelled reagents to give enhanced sensitivity. Improvements to instrumentation also help to improve sensitivity, as shown by the use of neon-helium lasers in nephelometers.

The introduction of instruments for more discriminating measurements, e.g. time-delayed fluorescence, particularly through the use of microprocessor controlled manipulation, will undoubtedly help realise the full potential of some techniques.

Conclusion

Immunoassays have played, and will continue to play, a major role in the quantitation of many analytes. There is every indication that the number and variety of applications will increase dramatically as the potential of this type of assay is appreciated in other areas. Two aspects invariably control the general development of any technique. One is the supply of suitable reagents, and the other is the introduction of practical instrumentation. The exploitation of monoclonal antibodies or affinity-purified antibodies will undoubtedly help assure provision of good reagents. Thus, it is apparent that development of instrumentation is an integral part of the further use of immunoassay methods. It is undoubtedly the critical factor when considering the major applications.

Further Reading

Langone J.J., Van Vunakis H., eds. (1982). *Methods in Enzymology, Vol. 84: Immunochemical Techniques, Part D.* London: Academic Press.

Parratt D., McKenzie H., Nielsen K.H., Cobb S.J. (1982). *Radioimmunoassay of Antibody and its Clinical Applications.* New York: John Wiley & Sons.

Voller A., Bartlett A., Bidwell D. (1981). *Immunoassays for the 80s.* Lancaster: MTP Press.

Voller A., Bidwell D., Bartlett A. (1979). *The Enzyme Linked Immunosorbent Assay (ELISA),* Vols. 1 & 2. Nuffield Laboratories of Comparative Medicine.

Index

accuracy of assay, 21
acridinum esters, 105–6
acronyms, 1–2
affinity
  antibody–antigen, 21
  chromatography, 68–72
  constant *see* equilibrium constant
allergen measurement, 48–9
analyte
  concentrations, 139–40
  nature, 141–2
antibody
  characteristics, 20–1
  chromatographic purification, 68–72
  heterogeneity, 61
  molecular structure, 12–13
  monoclonal, 62–8
  purification, 45–6, 69–72
  radiolabelling, 46–7
  second, 34–5
antigen, 18
antisera
  antibody heterogeneity, 61
  development, 9
  testing, 58–61

applications of assay, 148–53
avidity, antibody, 20

bacterial plaque assays, 133–4
bioluminescence, 107
biphasic response, 52–3
Bolton and Hunter reagent, 31
bound fraction, 18

chemiluminescence, 101, 103–4
chromatography, antibody purification, 69–72
complement fixation assays, 132–3
concentration ranges, 139–40
conjugation labelling, 31
constant region, 13
contamination of monoclonal antibodies, 65
cost of assay, 147
crossed immunoelectrophoresis, 117–19

desalting technique, 32–3
DID *see* double immunodiffusion
direct haemagglutination immunoassay, 124
double immunodiffusion, 113–15

electroimmunoassay, 115–17
ELISA *see* enzyme-labelled immunosorbent assays
enhancement, 153–7
  fluoroimmunoassays, 90
enzyme
  choice, 80–2
  immunoassay, 74–5
  label preparation, 83–4
  labelled immunosorbent assays, 78
  linked immunosorbent assay, 79–80
equilibrium, constant, 21–2

FETI *see* fluorescent excitation transfer fluoroimmunoassay
FIA *see* fluorescent immunoassay
fluorescence, 87
  protection immunoassay, 92
fluorescent excitation transfer fluoroimmunoassay, 94
fluorimetry, 98–9
fluoroimmunoassay
  enhancement, 90
  excitation, 94
  heterogeneous, 94
  homogeneous, 95
  polarisation, 89
  quenching, 90–2
fluorophores, 88
  choice, 96–8
FPIA *see* fluorescence protection immunoassay
free fraction, 18

gamma counter, 27

haemagglutination, 124–31
  inhibition immunoassay, 129
haemolysis immunoassays, 131–3
hapten principle, 58
heterogeneous fluoroimmunoassays, 94–5
homogeneous assays, 75–7
immunofluorometric assay, 95
'hook' effect *see* biphasic response

IFMA *see* immunofluorimetric assays
immune response, 55
immunisation, 57–8, 72
immunoassay methods, 13–16
immunodiffusion, 113–15
immunoelectrophoresis, 115–19
immunofluorometric assays, 95–6
immunogen, 56–7
immunometric assay, 16–18
immunoprecipitation, 34–5, 119

methods, 121
immunoprecipitates, 72
immunoradiometric assay, 40–53
indirect
  haemagglutination, 124–8
  labelling, 42–3
inhibition nephelometry, 122
Iodine-125 *see* radioiodine
IRMA *see* immunoradiometric assays
isoluminol and derivatives, 104–5

K *see* equilibrium constant

labelled
  antibody, 78
  reagents, 8
labels, 18–20
  bioluminescent, 107–8
  enzyme, 78–84
  fluorescent, 88–9
  indirect, 42–4
  luminescent, 100–10
  non-specific binding, 51
  radioactive, 25–36
latex
  nephelometry, 123, 136
  particle immunoassay, 134–7
LEIA *see* luminescent enzyme immunoassay
light scattering immunoassay, 120
luminescence, 100
luminescent
  enzyme immunoassay, 106
  reactions, 100–2

luminometry, 102
lymphocyte fusion, 62, 64

microtitre plate, 82–3
monoclonal antibodies, 62–8
multi-well gamma counter, 38

nephelometry, 120–23
non-specific binding of labels, 51–2

PACIA *see* particle counting immunoassay
particle counting immunoassay, 137
passive
  haemagglutination, 124–8
  haemolysis inhibition assay, 132
peroxidase-labelled conjugates, 106
PHI *see* passive haemolysis inhibition assay
polarisation fluoroimmunoassay, 89
polyethylene glycol, 35
precipitation, 111
precipitin test, 111–3
precision profiles, 50–1
'prozone' effect *see* biphasic response
purification
  antibodies, 45–6, 68–72
  radiolabels, 32–3

quantitation of fractions, 18–20
quenching
  fluoroimmunoassay, 90–2

radioallergosorbent test, 47–9
radioimmunoassay
  advantages, 2
  performance, 37–8
  separation techniques, 33–4
radioiodine
  incorporation, 28
  labels, 26–30
radioisotopes, 24–6
  half-life, 37
  hazards, 37
radiolabelling antibodies, 46–7
range
  of assays, 140–1
  of concentrations, 139–40
RAST *see* radioallergosorbent test
reagent
  availability, 144–5
  excess, 16–18
  fluorescent, 88
  kits, 10–11
  labelled, 8
  limited amount, 15–16, 74
  quality, 144–5
  sequential addition, 44–5
  solid-phase, 10, 35
  unlabelled, 8
reverse passive haemagglutination, 129–30
RIA *see* radioimmunoassay
rocket immunoelectrophoresis, 115–17
rosetting reaction assays, 134

sample type, 143
saturation analysis, 7
second antibody, 34–5
sensitivity
  immunoradiometric assay, 49
  radioimmunoassay, 3
sequential addition of reagents, 44–5
simplicity, radioimmunoassay, 5
single radial immunodiffusion, 113
solid-phase
  reagent, 10, 35–6
  separation techniques, 40–41
specificity
  antibody, 20
  immunoradiometric assay, 49
  monoclonal antibodies, 65
  radioimmunoassay, 5
SRID *see* single radial immunodiffusion
Stokes shift, 87

technical complexity, 145–7
test parameters, 143–4
time resolved fluorimetry, 98–9
titration, antisera, 59
titre, antibody, 20
turbidimetry, 121–3
  latex particle, 136–7
two-site immunometric method, 41–2

universal application, 6
unlabelled reagents, 8

valency, antibody, 20
variable region, 13